BMA

FAMILY DOCTOR GUIDES

Confusion in Old Age

Dr J. P. Wattis

Series editor: Dr Tony Smith

Dr Wattis is consultant in the psychiatry of old age at St James's Hospital, Leeds

EQUATION

Published by Equation in association with the British Medical Association

First published 1988

British Library Cataloguing in Publication Data

Wattis, John
Confusion in old age.
1. Old persons. Mental disorders
I. Title   II. Series
618.97'689

ISBN 1-85336-076-7

Picture acknowledgements
John Rae: pp. 7, 25, 26, 45, 53, 59, 61, 67, 71, 91; Geriatric
Medicine: pp. 11, 42, 86; Age Concern: pp. 21, 22, 34, 104; MRC
Cyclotron unit, Hammersmith Hospital: p. 37; Optical Information
Council: p. 57; Nursing Times: p. 77; David Woodroffe: diagrams;
Derek Marriott: cartoons.

Typeset by Columns of Reading
Printed and bound in Great Britain
by The Bath Press, Avon.

Equation, Wellingborough, Northamptonshire NN8 2RQ, England.

10 9 8 7 6 5 4 3 2 1

Contents

1 Introduction

When elderly people become confused, we describe them as getting 'senile'. It is as though we think that all old people are bound to suffer some loss of their mental abilities. This is not true. Most old people, even those who live to great old age, do not suffer any important loss in mental ability except perhaps in the last few weeks before death. A small number, however, do become confused, either temporarily as a result of a physical illness or some other stress in their life, or permanently because of one of the dementing illnesses. Temporary confusion and dementia are not the same.

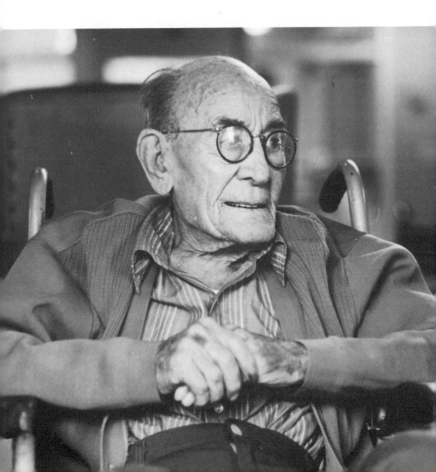

This book is mainly about the illnesses that cause dementia but it also considers other conditions that can be mistaken for dementia. The dementing illnesses cause progressive damage to memory, orientation, reasoning ability, and personality, and most cannot be directly treated medically (though there are a few exceptions). But even when there is no cure for the disease itself, medical, psychological, and social help will often improve the quality of life for both sufferers and carers.

Helping carers

This booklet aims to help those involved in the care of demented old people. It explains the various forms of confusion and dementia, the treatments available and how to find your way around the medical, social, legal, and financial services provided by the state and private and voluntary agencies.

2 Social effects of dementia

The impact of dementia on the sufferer can be devastating. Previously intelligent and responsible people may be unable to manage their own money, keep the house tidy, or even keep themselves clean. They may lose all sense of time so that they get up in the middle of the night to go to a job they have not worked in for many years. They may fail to recognise their homes or even their spouses. They may forget where they have put things and, in an attempt to make sense of what is happening, accuse others of stealing them. The ability to distinguish right and left or put clothes on in the right order may be lost.

Inappropriate behaviour

Sometimes they may persist with tasks that are inappropriate or no longer relevant. This may mean that they repeat a present task – for example, putting on several layers of clothes in the middle of summer. Alternatively they may undertake some task, perhaps one they used at work, in an inappropriate way or at an odd time. One woman, for example, often found her demented mother sewing. If not watched she would sew the hem of her dress to the sleeve so the daughter took to providing scraps of material for the old lady to work on.

Old people may cross the road without looking

9

Dangerous behaviour

Sufferers may do things that are a danger to themselves or others. They may leave the gas on unlit, burn pans, burn clothes, cross the road without looking, wander out in the middle of the night and get lost, or eat mouldy food. Sufferers often don't realise what they are doing – they don't remember their dangerous behaviour and deny the need for help. This can be very frustrating for you particularly if other people are 'taken in'. And loss of judgement can make sufferers easy game for unscrupulous criminals.

This lack of judgement and insight can make life less traumatic for sufferers, who may be blissfully unaware of the mess they are in, but it often causes major problems for carers, who may be unable to persuade them that any help is needed.

Impact on carers

Close relatives, especially children and spouses, find it hard to adjust to the new roles demanded of them.

- The wife of one demented old man found it particularly hard to make decisions. Before her husband was ill he used to take all the decisions and this worked well. He was a well qualified and intelligent man and she was devastated by the change in him.
- Another wife, in a similar position, had always had more say in household affairs and managed better. She was particularly distressed because her husband still had some insight and although he was quite severely demented, at times there were flashes of his old intelligence and quick wit. Despite a lot of support she was worn down by the 24 hour task of looking after him.
- One old man with a severely demented wife cared for her dilligently, helping her with washing and going to the toilet. The last straw for him was when she failed to recognise him, and believing him to be a stranger, started to resist his attempts to help.
- A pensioner, who was crippled by arthritis, still managed to care for his severely demented wife. The situation only broke down when she locked him out of the house. He had to climb in through a window and this caused such a severe attack of arthritis that they both had to go into hospital for a time.

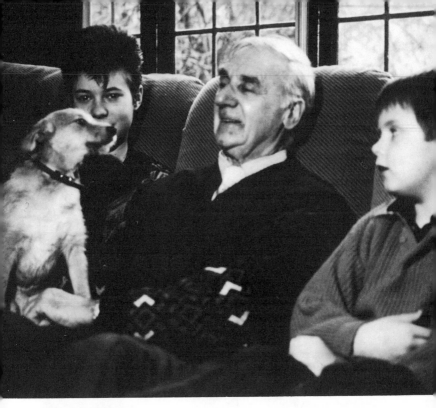

Families do care

Sometimes children take a demented parent into their own home but as the disability increases they find themselves unable to cope with the 24 hour supervision needed. The burden of caring conflicts with other equally important demands on time and energy such as the needs of other family members or the need to earn a living. The idea that present day families do not care for old people is quite false. Many relatives provide care and supervision far beyond what could reasonably be expected and it should be one of the priorities of the health and social services to provide support to these carers. Without them the situation would indeed be desperate.

> **Without carers, the situation for many old people would be desperate.**

'Living bereavement'

Apart from the practical difficulties of coping with a close relative who needs more or less constant supervision, sufferers' relatives also have to cope with the emotional burden. After bereavement people pass through a process of grieving in which numbness is followed by sorrow, often mingled with anger at the loss. Learning to cope with the grief takes months, and sometimes years. Late in the grieving process, it is important to fill the gaps in life left by the dead person. When a relative develops severe dementia it is, in some respects, as if he or she has died. The unaffected partner experiences a kind of bereavement but far from being able to resolve the grief, is constantly reminded, by the sufferer's presence, of the relationship they used to share. Nor is there any opportunity to fill the gaps in life, the partner often demands and needs ever increasing care and attention. This process and experience has been called 'living bereavement'.

> **Taking care of a severely demented husband or wife can be harder than losing them through death.**

Stresses of caring

People who have lost a loved one through death sometimes experience grief in a way that makes life more difficult than it need be. Similar reactions may be seen in the relatives of dementia sufferers. They may try to deny what is happening, claiming that the sufferer is just 'a bit forgetful' and hiding the seriousness of the problem from themselves, their friends, and the helping services. Others may become angry at God, the medical profession, or the social services for their misfortune. Occasionally this anger may spill over into mistreatment of the sufferer especially if the family is one in which physical violence has been a common reaction to stress. Couples who have worked hard all their lives and looked forward to a shared retirement may suddenly find their plans ruined by dementia. People often ask, 'Why us?' Sometimes relatives can become very bitter. The combination of the emotional stresses of 'living bereavement' and practical stresses such as providing constant supervision despite sleepless nights, can lead to the carer becoming extremely anxious or depressed, so that they need medical or psychological treatment.

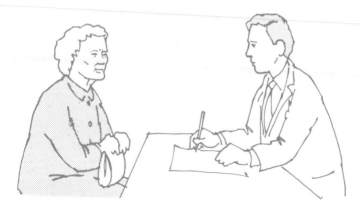

The combination of emotional and practical stresses of caring for someone who is demented can lead to severe anxiety or depression that needs medical treatment.

Mrs Roberts was an 80 year old who had always had very high standards and, with her husband, had been a respected member of her local church.

Unfortunately, Mr Roberts developed dementia. Mrs Roberts found it very hard to accept that anything was wrong, even when her husband needed help with dressing and keeping clean. She felt 'duty bound' to take him out but at the same time was ashamed of the man she had once been proud of. Her reluctance to admit to the outside world that he was ill, her sense of duty, and the fact that her husband was upset when she was not around all made it hard for her to accept day care help, which would have been one way of relieving the constant strain.

Gradually, Mrs Roberts became more and more depressed, despite regular visits to the psychiatrist for support and drug treatment. She still would not agree to day care or periods of residential care for her husband. Eventually she became so depressed that she was thinking of suicide.

She was finally persuaded that her husband should go in to residential care so that she could come into hospital for treatment. In hospital, and with treatment, her depression lifted. She continued to feel guilty about her husband being in residential care, however, and when she went home, insisted that he should return too. She was prepared, however, to allow a limited amount of day care for him. Mrs Roberts is still visited by a community nurse and attends a hospital clinic as her depression has returned, but she is not so severely affected as before.

Mutual support

Carers often find comfort in sharing their problems with others in a similar situation. Mutual support groups may be run by local social services, psychiatric services, or voluntary groups. The usefulness of these groups in helping you to cope with the emotional burden of caring for a dementia sufferer cannot be over emphasised. Some groups run for a fixed number of sessions, others are continuous. Usually they combine a short talk from an expert on some aspect of caring for dementia sufferers with a session for mutual discussion of problems, often over a cup of tea or coffee. If arrangements need to be made for your demented relative to be cared for during the session, some groups can provide a substitute carer. Telephone advice services, run by groups like Alzheimer's Disease Society or Age Concern are also developing. Your family doctor, social worker, or the national parent organisations will be able to tell you if there is a group near you. (There are useful phone numbers on p.101)

A national challenge

Not much over a hundred years ago nearly half of all children born in some parts of the UK died before their 6th birthday. In other parts of the world this situation still exists. Here, medical advances, especially improved sanitation, have led to a dramatic reduction in infant deaths and now most people will only face death in old age.

More old people and fewer carers

People over the age of 65 formed only about 5% of the total UK population in 1900; now they form around 15%. More importantly, in terms of our present concern, the number and proportion of very old people is increasing, and it is these people who are most at risk of developing dementia. They are also more likely to have a variety of medical problems and suffer certain social disadvantages (for example, half the women over the age of 75 live alone). The ratio of middle aged people (potential caregivers) to people over the age of 75 has dropped from around 10 to one in 1931 to around three to one now. Geographical mobility and the fact that many more women go out to work have also contributed to a reduction in the number of potential supporters available to the very aged.

Old people as a percentage of the total population (UK)

	Over 65	75–84 years	85 years and over
1901	4.7	1.2	0.2
1951	11.0	3.1	0.5
1981	15.1	4.8	1.0
2001	14.3	5.0	1.5

Source: Adapted from *Dementia in Old Age*, Office of Health Economics, London.

Percentage of dementia sufferers in relation to age

Age	Percentage
65–69	2
70–74	3
75–79	6
80 +	22

Source: Kay, Bergman, McKechnie and Roth (1970).

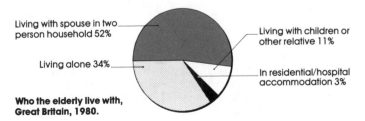

Living with spouse in two person household 52%

Living with children or other relative 11%

Living alone 34%

In residential/hospital accommodation 3%

Who the elderly live with, Great Britain, 1980.

Effects on the NHS

Perhaps 2% of old people are in hospital beds, but between them they occupy nearly 50% of those beds. Again, the very old are more likely to need hospital or residential care than younger members of society. Although Britain has the second most aged population in the world and despite the fact that our old people need more health and social services care than other groups, we spend less on health care than most other developed nations. This is one of the main reasons behind the recurrent financial crises of the National Health Service. Unusually low spending against a background of unusually high needs is bound to create problems.

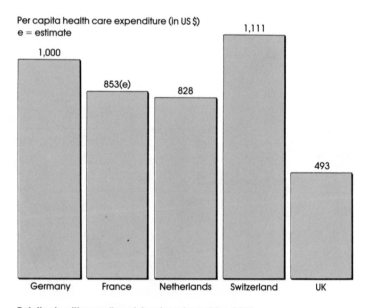

Per capita health care expenditure (in US $)
e = estimate

Relative health spending of developed countries, 1982.

Despite the shortage of resources, however, psychiatric and medical services for old people in this country are still regarded as world leaders in some respects, especially the emphasis on assessment of their needs and community care. This is partly due to the fact that the centralised planning of the

NHS has led to the development of specialised services for old people. About two thirds of old people live in areas where they can be referred to specialised psychiatric services that can provide help in the diagnosis and management of dementia and other mental illnesses.

Setting the background

This booklet will concentrate on the underlying causes of confusion, from the dementing illnesses through the impact of other mental and physical illnesses (including loss of hearing and eyesight) to the effect of the surroundings on the confused old person. In the next chapter, however, we will step back from the problems of ageing and set the background by looking at normal old age.

3 What is normal in old age

Many of the changes of old age can be easily seen. Shakespeare ruthlessly parodies the changes of extreme old age in his lines from *As You Like It*.

> . . . The sixth age shifts
> Into the lean and slipper'd pantaloon,
> With spectacles on nose and pouch on side,
> His youthful hose well sav'd a world too wide
> For his shrunk shank; and his big manly voice,
> Turning again towards childish treble, pipes
> And whistles in his sound. Last scene of all
> That ends this strange eventful history,
> Is second childishness and mere oblivion,
> Sans teeth, sans eyes, sans taste, sans everything.

Not all changes are inevitable

Like many observers Shakespeare confuses the changes that are to be expected in old age, such as some loss of muscle tissue ('his shrunk shank') with others that are by no means inevitable ('second childishness'). It is important to distinguish between changes that are evident in almost all old people and so can be seen as a part of 'normal' ageing and those that are the result of specific illnesses. The latter changes, though more common in old people, are by no means 'normal' and are not dealt with here. In this chapter, we will consider the changes in the body (physical changes) that occur with increasing age and then in more detail some of the psychological changes of ageing. Relevant social changes will also be mentioned.

18

Physical changes

The body can be viewed as a group of interlocking systems that provide support to the brain. The gastro-intestinal system (stomach and intestines) extracts energy and nutrients from food and gets rid of waste matter. In old age it does not suffer many changes, though constipation probably becomes more common – perhaps as a result of reduced exercise and, in some cases, of a poor diet. The liver (which stores and processes nutrients) also becomes less efficient in tasks like breaking down alcohol and certain medicines. This and other changes mean that old people are often more susceptible to the effects of alcohol and medications, whether prescribed by doctors or bought 'over the counter' from the chemist.

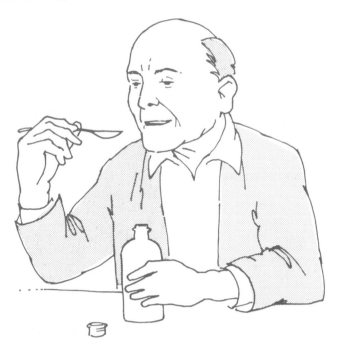

Old people are often more susceptible to the effects of medicines.

19

Heart and blood vessels

The cardio-vascular system (heart and blood vessels) becomes less efficient. Fatty tissues can be deposited in the walls of blood vessels, especially in men, and this is a common cause of heart attacks and strokes. Strictly speaking this is not a 'normal' change since it is related to diet and smoking. Nevertheless it is so common in Western societies at present that it is included here. For other reasons too, the cardio-vascular system has less 'reserve' in old age and can more easily fail because of illness in other body systems.

> **Eating a sensible diet which is low in fat and not smoking can help protect against diseases of the heart and blood vessels.**

Lungs

The respiratory system (airways and lungs) also often has less reserve in old age. Again this is partly an effect of age itself but can be made worse by smoking and repeated chest infections. The respiratory and the cardio-vascular systems are closely connected and failure in one readily leads to problems in the other.

Genito-urinary system

The genito-urinary system suffers many changes with age. In women the ability to have children stops at the menopause and this brings with it changes in hormones that can lead to thinning of the bones (osteoporosis) and a greater likelihood of suffering fractures. There is some evidence to suggest that exercise before the menopause can help to protect against this by building stronger bones. In some women hormone replacement therapy or supplements of calcium (vital for strong bones) may be needed but these, especially hormone replacement treatment, are not entirely without risk and so are not given routinely. In men, the ability to father children is often retained into old age but the prostate gland sometimes gives trouble, making it difficult to pass urine.

The kidneys, which are in effect filtering and processing systems to purify the blood and get rid of waste, may be less efficient and have less reserve. This can influence the body's ability to cope with some medications. Some old people experience physical changes that affect their ability to control their bladder.

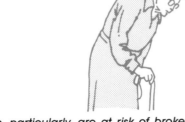

Women, particularly, are at risk of broken bones as they get older.

Muscles and bones

As suggested by Shakespeare, the muscular part of the musculo-skeletal system tends to be reduced and as we age we carry proportionately more fat. As well as affecting strength and endurance in physical tasks, these changes, by altering the proportion of water in the body, can also increase the effects that alcohol and certain medications have on us. In women especially, thinning of the bones can make broken bones more likely. Regular, reasonable exercise can help

Regular, reasonable exercise can help.

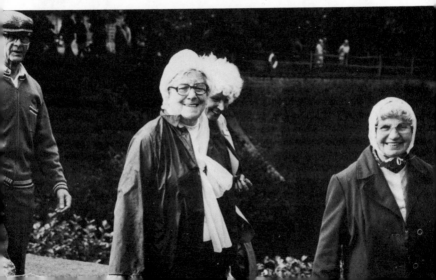

reduce the loss of muscle bulk as well as keeping the heart and lungs healthy. Overweight people (and those who have taken certain forms of violent exercise, such as rugby) are more prone to develop wear and tear diseases of the joints (osteoarthritis) in later life.

Nervous system

The nervous system may become less able to react to extremes of temperature so that some old people are prone to hypothermia and (less often in this country!) heat stroke. Sometimes the nervous system's ability to regulate blood pressure on standing up can be reduced too. This problem can be made worse by some medications, and this may lead to a tendency to faint when standing up suddenly.

Hearing and vision

Hearing and vision are sometimes reduced by ageing changes, and sometimes by treatable disease.

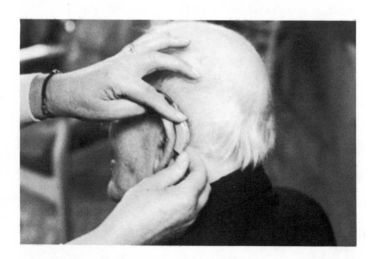

Less protection

The immune system, which helps protect us from disease, may not always be able to cope so well with infections as it can in younger people.

Not a catalogue of despair

This may sound like a catalogue of despair but it is important to remember that in most old people the changes described are relatively minor and amount to a loss of reserve capacity rather than a complete loss of function. Many of the changes can be reduced or prevented by a sensible lifestyle – restricting alcohol, exercising in moderation, and avoiding smoking and fatty foods. Other changes are due to disease and in some cases can be prevented by medical treatment. Changes in hearing or vision can sometimes be treated medically and often compensated for by the use of hearing aids and spectacles. When, in the next chapter, we discuss the interactions between our mental and physical functions, you will see why it is so important to maintain maximum fitness in these other systems.

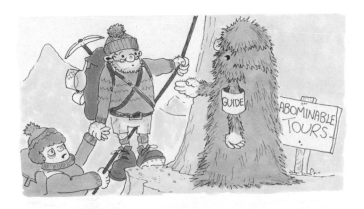

Psychological changes

Some psychological changes such as a slowing in the time it takes to react to an outside event are the result of changes in the brain and nervous system. Like other organs, the brain often seems to have a reduction in reserve capacity with increasing age. Inevitably, some nerve cells die but most people still have enough to carry on functioning perfectly normally. The brain probably shrinks a little as we age and there are slight reductions in the number of neurotransmitters that act as chemical messengers between nerve cells.

A decline in intelligence?

Certain researchers have suggested that there is a decline of intelligence with old age. The studies on which these ideas were originally based were flawed in that they compared old and young people of different generations with different educational backgrounds. More recent studies, which have followed people as they age, suggest that any changes in intellect that occur in normal ageing are minimal. The ability to solve new problems in psychological brain teasers may be slightly reduced, but in everyday life this is probably more than compensated for by the increasing wisdom of experience. In fact, in psychological testing there are some tasks which a young child can perform more efficiently than a teenager or young adult but we do not normally speak of a decline in intelligence between childhood and teenage!

Do we become more fixed?

Studies which have found personality becomes more 'rigid' with increasing age have probably been biased by the accidental inclusion of people with mental illnesses (including early dementia), which are increasingly common with advancing years. Personality certainly develops with increasing age and most of us recognise that we are not quite the same person we were 10 to 20 years ago. Experience changes our attitudes and our habitual ways of reacting to life. People who are rigid, overbearing, or excessively dependent may certainly become more so as they increase in age; but given the right circumstances and friends, the opposite may well happen.

Social changes

Retirement is one of the most important social changes for many people. Those who have been dependent on their work for status and friends may be particularly hard hit. Many firms are now running pre-retirement courses to help their employees cope with this transition. In some states of the USA, a different approach has been taken. It has been said that forcing people to retire on grounds of age alone is a form of discrimination ('ageism') and compulsory retirement on these grounds has been made illegal. Certainly, people should be given the option to retire later as well as earlier if they are still competent at their job.

Not so well off

People are often less well off financially when they retire. The loss of income from work makes a particular impact on those who do not have much in the way of savings or an occupational pension, but those who have been earning reasonable wages can cushion themselves against the financial impact of retirement by investing in appropriate savings and pension schemes.

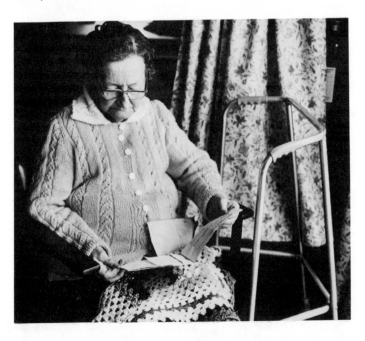

Some move house

Old people are affected by geographical migration. In some areas the old people themselves move into a particular area (for example, the South Coast) at retirement. In other areas, such as inner cities and rural areas they tend to be left behind, often in substandard property, as the younger people move to the suburbs of the big cities and towns. This can result in areas where there are large numbers of old people, making help from younger relatives more difficult and throwing an extra burden on the health and social services.

Difficulties with transport

Isolation can often be made worse by loss of a car, either as a result of disability or because of poverty. Old people often rely on public transport and are particularly vulnerable to cuts in provision.

Losing loved ones

Bereavement adds to the social and psychological stress of growing old.

Advantages of retirement

On the other hand, there are many advantages in retirement and many people adapt well to a new life style and new roles as grandparents and even great grandparents. People can take up or expand a hobby or may even take up a 'second career' by going for further education or getting involved in voluntary work. There is great scope for a positive attitude towards making more use of the greatly under utilised resources of experience, skills, and abilities of old people.

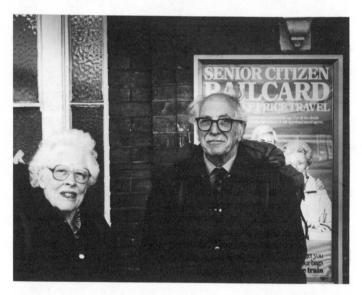

Some people set out on new adventures when they retire.

4 Understanding confusion

Doctors use the term 'confusion' to describe a symptom, and a symptom may be a pointer to a whole range of possible diseases. It is particularly important to remember this when we are dealing with 'confusion'. All too often the wrong assumption may be made that confusion is necessarily caused by dementia (or 'senility') and that nothing can therefore be done about it. If confusion is regarded as a pointer to the possibility of many different causes, then these can be considered in a logical way, and even where there is dementia, commonsense ways may be found to reduce the confusion.

Four elements in confusion

One of the simplest ways to consider the different causes of confusion is illustrated on p. 31. This starts at the centre with the brain, then considers factors in the physical supporting systems that may be important. The special senses, particularly hearing and vision, form the interface with the outside world and damage to those can contribute to confusion. Finally, factors in our surroundings can also help produce confusion.

The brain

The brain is a very complicated system that stores all that we have ever learned in life. Things like personality and intelligence are largely a function of the brain. Even our spiritual hopes and beliefs cannot be expressed independently of the brain. When we consider confusion, it is important to think of how previous personality traits and ways of coping with stress will influence the form it takes.

The main causes of confusion

With the structure of the brain, the main causes of confusion in old age are two diseases – Alzheimer's disease and multi-infarct (or arteriosclerotic) dementia. The brain may also be

Miss Long lived in a block of flats. She had led a very interesting life, running a women's hostel in London during the 'blitz'. She had always been a very lively person who had high expectations of herself and others and was used to being 'in charge'.

In her late 70s, Miss Long slowly developed memory impairment. She also began to worry that other people in the block were trying to get her out of her flat because it was wanted for a married couple. (Whether this represented an imperfect memory of some event earlier in her life, we were unable to determine.) At the same time, she also believed that the block was a girls' hostel and that she was somehow 'in charge' of it and responsible for cooking for the girls!

As her condition deteriorated, she started to neglect herself but it was impossible to persuade her to consider residential or even day care because she was worried about what would happen to 'my girls'. She had some arguments with other people in the flats who denied any intention to force her out and did not admit to the authority which she believed was hers! Eventually Miss Long collapsed and had to be admitted to hospital.

After recovery, she was not really well enough to live in her own home, even with maximum social support. Subsequently this lady was settled in residential care.

damaged by repeated injury (boxers are sometimes affected), poisonous substances (including alcohol), and physical diseases such as untreated thyroid and some vitamin deficiencies. If caught at an early stage, the dementias caused by alcohol and thyroid or vitamin deficiency can sometimes be reversed or at least stopped by appropriate medical treatment. The structural changes, particularly of Alzheimer's disease, are accompanied by biochemical deficiencies in neurotransmitters (the chemical messengers between nerve cells) however, and cannot be reversed. Other diseases such as depressive illness and schizophrenia can produce biochemical changes without much structural damage. In old age they can sometimes look like confusion and be mistaken for dementia. This is a serious mistake since depressive illness and schizophrenia respond well to medical treatment.

> In the brain, the main causes of confusion in old age are • Alzheimer's disease, • multi-infarct dementia, • repeated injury, • excessive alcohol consumption, • vitamin or thyroid deficiencies, • mental illnesses such as depression or schizophrenia.

The body

All the losses of reserves in different body systems described in the previous chapter mean that an illness in one system can easily lead to problems in other systems. When this occurs, the brain may be suddenly unable to cope with all the changes in its support systems and an 'acute confusional state' results.

The senses

During the process of 'brainwashing' sometimes used to extract 'confessions' from prisoners, a commonly used technique is that of sensory deprivation. In experiments volunteers submitted to total sensory deprivation by being subjected to silence, darkness, and sometimes insulated from touch, quickly become confused, experience hallucinations, and become suggestible so that they accept new ideas relatively uncritically. Many old people, while not being subject to total sensory deprivation, may not be able to see or hear very well, which makes it harder for them to make sense of what is going on around them and may lead to confusion.

The surroundings

Another way of causing confusion is to put someone through a series of rapid changes in their surroundings. When old people who are already ill are admitted to hospital in an emergency, this is often exactly what happens to them and if care is not taken to make sure they know what is happening any confusion they already have can easily be worsened.

Managing change properly is vitally important for those old people who are already a bit confused. The surroundings can be used to help. We are all familiar with the use of a shopping list and other memory aids. For old people with early dementia there are often many practical ways of using reminders to assist them to make full use of their remaining abilities.

Interactions

The most important thing about this way of looking at confusion is that it is *interactive* – factors work together or singly to produce confusion. In one person confusion may be entirely due to brain disease. In another there may be little or no brain disease but a combination of physical illness and the environmental change of hospital admission may produce a similar, though temporary, degree of confusion. Impaired hearing or eyesight may make it much harder for sufferers to appreciate what is going on around them, adding to confusion, and unsympathetic or hurried handling from hospital staff may have a similar effect.

A positive approach

When confusion is regarded in this way, the defeatist attitude that confusion is always caused by irreversible brain disease alone can be avoided. And it is worth emphasising again that even when dementia is present, other factors such as poor hearing or eyesight or physical ill health, may make the problem worse than it needs be and sometimes these other problems will respond to medical treatment. Changes can also be made in the environment to compensate for failing memory. The simplest examples are lists or notes to remind sufferers what to do next and clearly marked (or even colour coded) toilet areas in day centres or other facilities used by confused people.

More detail

Having briefly considered the various contributions to causing the symptom of confusion, we will go on in succeeding chapters to consider each contribution in more detail.

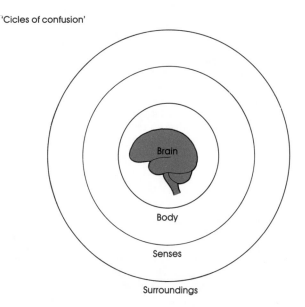

'Cicles of confusion'

Brain

Body

Senses

Surroundings

Four elements of confusion

5 Confusion—
dementing illnesses

Alzheimer's disease is by far the commonest cause of dementia. It accounts for well over half of all dementias in old age. Up to another fifth of dementias are due to vascular disease. These are often referred to as arteriosclerotic or multi-infarct dementia. Perhaps another fifth are due to a mixture of Alzheimer's disease and multi-infarct dementia and the remainder are the result of a variety other causes. Alcohol probably contributes to more dementias in old age than is generally recognised, either directly through a toxic effect on the brain or indirectly through vitamin deficiencies that excessive drinking causes. Since drinking too much alcohol also tends to cause increased blood pressure and since there is a link between increased blood pressure and multi- infarct dementia, alcohol may also contribute to some cases of this. Other, relatively rare causes of dementia in old age include vitamin B12 and thyroid deficiency. Sometimes a slow growing brain tumour or clot of blood on the brain can produce confusion. There also seems to be a slight link between Parkinson's disease and dementia.

More unusual causes

Very rarely, dementia may be the result of a late stage of syphilis. Now, though not in old people yet, we are beginning to see dementia as a result of the acquired immune deficiency syndrome (AIDS). Among young people, dementia of all types is uncommon but when it does occur Alzheimer's disease or multi-infarct dementia are often the cause. Other causes of dementia in younger people are Pick's disease where the front part of the brain, which controls social behaviour, is often affected first, and Huntingdon's chorea, a very rare inherited disorder where abnormal movements and other psychiatric symptoms often come before the dementia. Here, there will only be space to consider Alzheimer's disease and multi-infarct dementia in detail.

Alzheimer's disease

This is the form of dementia most often confused with ordinary ageing. This is because it comes on so slowly that at first it may be dismissed as ordinary forgetfulness. Relatives may be unable to put a finger on when the memory loss first began but eventually it reaches a pitch where things are clearly abnormal. Door keys and purses are persistently mislaid, the sufferer becomes uncertain about what time of day or what day of the week it is. The problem may first come to light when the sufferer goes on holiday and gets lost and confused in unfamiliar surroundings. Eventually they may get lost in their own neighbourhood or even in their own house. Sometimes they may believe that they are not even at home, giving a childhood address instead of their present one. Sufferers may fail to recognise acquaintances and eventually even their own spouses or children.

No sense of time

Loss of time sense occurs relatively early in the course of the disease and can be responsible for many problems, especially for people living alone. The sufferer may go for his or her pension in the middle of the night or on the wrong day. If he or she is living with a relative, night time wandering can also be a great irritation, though this can often be reduced by increased activity and stimulation during the day, by avoiding stimulant drinks (such as tea or coffee) and alcohol in the evening, and sometimes by medication, though this is best used only as a last resort.

Up to 800 000 people in this country have dementia, mostly Alzheimer's disease.

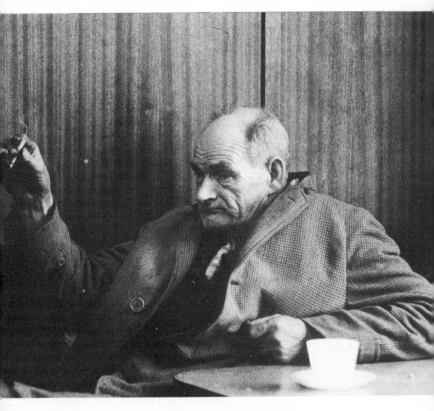

Personal hygiene suffers too.

Hygiene suffers too

The house may become neglected and dirty and eventually personal cleanliness suffers also. Generally these problems are much worse in people living alone. If they are with a spouse or children and have a relatively biddable personality then many of the problems mentioned above can be delayed by prompting and reminders. Eventually, however, the parts of the brain that enable recognition of items of clothing or the distinction between right and left may be affected so that the sufferer really cannot dress herself without a great deal of assistance.

34

Incontinence

Incontinence can occur because sufferers forget they need to go to the lavatory or forget where it is. At an early stage this can be managed by reminders to go to the toilet, if necessary showing the way. Later on, incontinence may be caused by restlessness (sometimes the result of constipation) and a failure to recognise the toilet. Sometimes special training or the use of medication to treat the constipation or control the restlessness can be of help. Rarely, nothing helps and the incontinence has to be accepted. In these cases, special incontinence pants, pads, and bed sheets can reduce the burden on carers. Most family doctors and district nurses can give help with these problems and for the more difficult patients, health districts usually have a continence adviser who can give expert assistance.

Special problems in residential homes

When people with dementia live in a residential home or long stay hospital, incontinence can often be inadvertently brought on by staff.

When staff numbers are too low – and, sadly, they often are – residents who are behaving themselves tend to get little attention. If, however, they are incontinent or 'misbehave' in some other way, then they get increased attention. Even if this is a 'scolding' it is still better than no attention and so the likelihood of the unwanted behaviour being repeated is increased. The answer to this problem is adequate numbers of trained staff, who can provide activities and attention for sufferers when they are behaving well rather than when some unwanted event such as incontinence occurs.

> **The understaffing of services for the elderly and particularly of many long stay hospital and residential facilities is a scandal which future generations may look back on with the same horror that we look back on child labour and slavery.**

How common is Alzheimer's disease?

Alzheimer's disease is very rare under the age of 65. From then on it becomes increasingly common with increasing age. For example, the rate between 65 and 70 is probably only 1 or 2% whereas over 80 the rate for dementia as a whole, which by this age is nearly all Alzheimer's disease, rises to more than 20%. To the optimist this means that even in extreme old age, four out of five people are *not* affected. To those charged with providing health and social services to old people against a background of restricted resources it is a frightening figure, however, since it is this very elderly age group who are expanding most rapidly. These overall figures for the prevalence of dementia can be misleading since there is increasing evidence that dementia may be slightly more common in some parts of the country than others.

Even in extreme old age only one out of every five people will suffer from dementia.

What causes Alzheimer's disease?

This question can be answered at two levels. Doctors have a fairly clear idea of the structural and chemical changes in the brain that are the immediate cause of the disease. Alzheimer (after whom this disorder is named) described the basic changes that could be seen under the microscope in the first decade of this century, and in the last 20 years it has been shown quite clearly that the amount of damage (called senile plaques and neurofibrillary tangles) corresponds to the severity of the dementia. In younger people the structural and chemical damage tends to be more widespread and the disease gets worse more quickly in this age group.

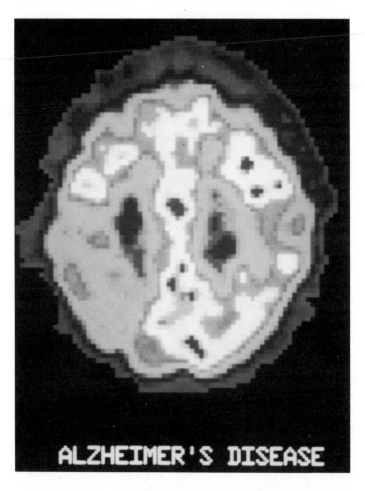

ALZHEIMER'S DISEASE

A PET scan of the brain of a patient with Alzheimer's disease showing reduced blood flow in several areas because cells are degenerating and not using as much energy as normal cells.

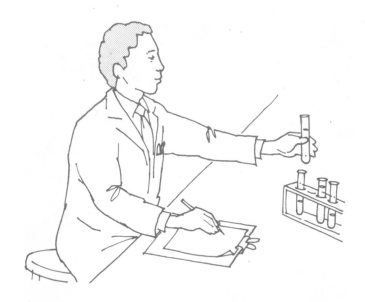

Chemical changes

In terms of chemical changes, the main substance involved is a chemical messenger between nerve and called acetylcholine. This substance is contained in nerve cells which normally, when activated, release it to activate the next nerve cell in the chain. Nerve cells which deal with memory are the main group to use acetylcholine in this way and it seems that in Alzheimer's disease these memory nerve cells are selectively destroyed. Because the receiving cells are left relatively intact, attempts have been made to treat sufferers with acetylcholine or a related substance, lecithin. Unfortunately, though tests have shown some nerve activity after treatment with these substances, they do not make enough difference for it to be worth using them as routine treatment. Other drugs act on this system and also seem to have some effects but it is too early yet to say whether these effects will be sufficient to help sufferers.

Many pharmaceutical companies are working hard to research medications that might work but even if they are successful, it will not yet mean a 'cure' for Alzheimer's disease. The problem is that we do not know how the nerve cells are damaged and killed and until we can identify and treat that process any treatment is likely to produce a temporary improvement only.

The underlying cause

Several ideas have been put forward to explain the underlying cause of Alzheimer's disease. Undoubtedly, in some families, particularly those where the disease affects relatively young members, a susceptibility to the disease (though *not* the disease itself) is inherited. It may be that exposure to something in the environment is then needed to trigger the disease. Two leading contenders for this role are an unusual virus or some chemical poison such as aluminium. Aluminium is a very common substance in the modern environment. It is, however, not normally well absorbed into the body or transferred from the blood to the brain if it does get into the body. Possibly it does get into the brain more easily in some people. Certainly it has recently been discovered at the core of senile plaques seen in the brain of those with Alzheimer's disease, though it is still not clear whether it is there as a cause of the problem or as accidental 'debris'.

Link with Down's syndrome

An interesting genetic link that has come to light recently is with Down's syndrome. People with this disease seem to be more likely than others to develop Alzheimer's disease at a relatively early stage of life and have the typical changes in the brain described earlier. Down's syndrome is related to an abnormality of one of the chromosomes, the basic genetic unit that carries all the hereditary material (genes) that makes us the people we are. There are 24 pairs of chromosomes in the cells of normal people. In Down's syndrome the chromosome given the number 21 is affected. Scientists now believe that they are close to finding the exact location of the gene on chromosome 21 that determines susceptibility to at least some forms of Alzheimer's disease.

Multi-infarct dementia

It is easiest to describe this form of dementia by contrasting it with Alzheimer's disease. Whereas Alzheimer's disease generally develops gradually multi-infarct dementia often starts with

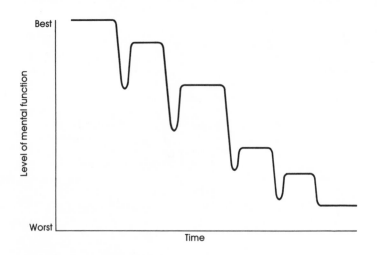

Multi-infant dementia time course.
(modified from Wattis and Church, p.71)

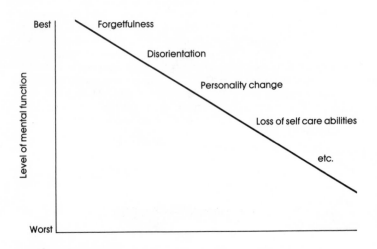

Alzheimer's disease time course.
(modified from Wattis and Church, p.71)

a sudden episode of confusion, perhaps associated with a stroke. After a partial recovery, the sufferer may remain relatively stable for a while until there is another episode of confusion, again with some recovery. The condition pursues what has been called a 'stepwise' course rather than the relatively smooth downhill course of Alzheimer's disease.

History of strokes

Patients with multi-infarct dementia often have a history of high blood pressure and may have a clear pattern of strokes affecting their physical abilities, though this is not always the case and not everyone who has several strokes develops this type of dementia. Because the disorder is caused by the death of small areas of brain after an obstruction to the blood supply, the clinical picture is often 'patchy' and the patient may still be able to function in some ways. Insight into their problem, mercifully rare in those with Alzheimer's disease, is not uncommon in patients with multi-infarct dementia, and they often suffer from depression (perhaps not surprisingly). Loss of control of the emotions is not infrequent either and may result in inappropriate weeping, anger, or, occasionally, laughter.

How common is multi-infarct dementia?

This dementia is certainly less common than Alzheimer's disease and may be becoming less common. It seems to be more frequent among men in their 60s and 70s and it appears that those things that predispose to stroke – high blood pressure and heart attack – may also be risk factors for multi-Infarct dementia. Thus smoking, excessive drinking, and obesity may have a part to play in causing this disease and this may explain why the disease seems to be becoming less common as we become more health conscious. Another factor in this may be the early detection and treatment of high blood pressure.

> **It is estimated that 160 000 people in Britain have multi-infarct dementia.**

What causes multi-infarct dementia?

Once it was believed that all dementia was due to 'hardening of the arteries'. This seems to be unlikely as an explanation for Alzheimer's disease, but for multi-infarct dementia it is probably the main cause. The modern term for hardening of the arteries is 'atherosclerosis'. In this condition, little areas of fatty material are deposited in the main blood vessels. Here they can either reduce the blood supply to the brain by partly obstructing the blood vessel or, more commonly, cause trouble by breaking off into the blood stream and being carried into smaller vessels. When this happens they sometimes plug the smaller vessel completely, cutting off the blood supply to a small area of brain. This is what causes the sudden episode of confusion and may cause an evident stroke.

The early detection and treatment of high blood pressure may help prevent multi-infarct dementia.

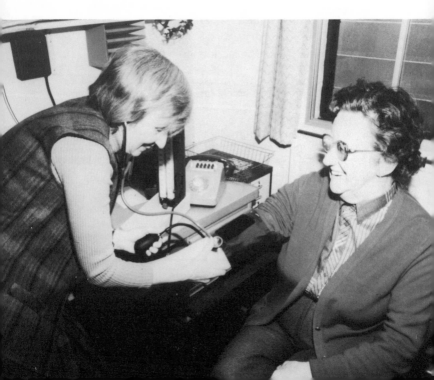

A more hopeful outlook

This difference from the unknown cause of Alzheimer's disease is important. Firstly, we know that atherosclerosis is, at least in part, a condition that can be prevented by leading a healthy lifestyle. Secondly, even after a stroke has occured, it may be that treatment designed to reduce the stickiness of the blood and thus the risk of further plugs blocking the small blood vessels can help slow the progression of the disease. The medication probably most often used for this purpose is a low dose of aspirin!

Conclusion

There are many possible causes of dementia in old age but Alzheimer's disease is by far the most common. Though we have discovered a great deal about this disease by scientific research we still do not know the underlying cause. The outlook for multi-infarct dementia, the second most common dementia in old age, is more optimistic. Here we have a clearer understanding of the underlying cause and so can offer advice on prevention. Also, although we cannot yet cure this disease, there is hope that research will discover medications which can prevent recurrent stroke and, by the same token, worsening of multi-infarct dementia. At present the humble aspirin in a very low dose (equivalent, to less than half a tablet a day) may have some small but considerable effect in slowing the progress.

6 Confusion – other mental illnesses

There are many different forms of nervous illness in old age. Partly because we expect old people to suffer from 'senility' these illnesses are too often confused with the dementias. This expectation is, however, only part of the reason. Many mental disorders in old age, especially severe depression, can cause the sufferer to become genuinely confused. This confusion must, however, be distinguished from the confusion found in dementia, since, provided the underlying cause is recognised, it responds well to medical treatment.

Depression

We all know what it's like to feel mildly depressed but the kind of depressive illness we are discussing here is something quite different. Sufferers from the severe forms of this disorder are unable to take pleasure in anything. Their appetite and weight are usually reduced and their sleep is often disturbed. They wake very early and usually feel particularly awful in the morning. Physical movements, thought processes, and even the bowels may be slowed down. Sometimes they will be agitated and restless, the same as some dementia sufferers. The worst aspects of the sufferer's previous personality may come to the fore. Demanding, dependent people become more demanding and dependent when they are depressed, insecure people more insecure and so on. There may be a serious risk of suicide.

What causes depression?

Severe depression may be triggered in susceptible people by major life stresses, especially bereavement. Often, but not always, sufferers will have had previous episodes of depression when they were young or other members of the family may have a history of depression. Depressive illness is often associated with physical ill health and may, of course, affect people who are suffering from dementia, thereby worsening their confusion.

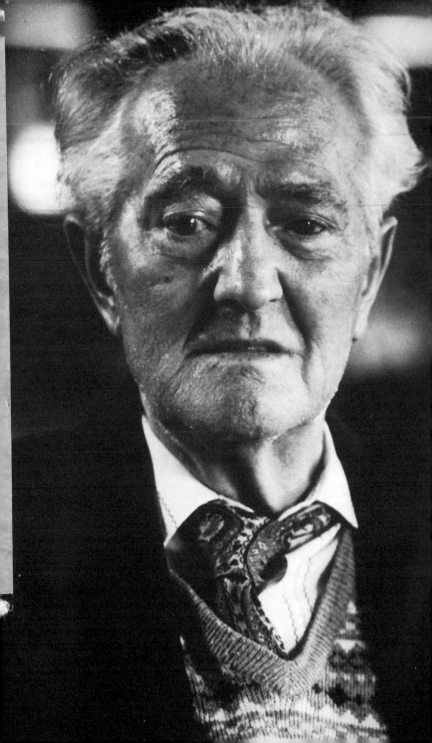

Depression can look like dementia

Severe depression may mimic dementia in several ways. Firstly, the slowing and agitation may interfere with memory and concentration so that the sufferer actually does have a (temporary) memory defect. Secondly, the depressed person may actually believe, as part of the depression, that he or she is useless and 'becoming senile'. In this situation the sufferer often gives answers that are vague or says, 'I don't know' to every question. These people are often very worried about their memory loss, unlike the typical Alzheimer's disease sufferer who, certainly in the later stages of the disease, is often blissfully unaware of the problem. Depression can also lead to confusion because of self-neglect resulting in nutritional deficiency, loss of body fluids, and other illness. Finally, some of the drugs used to treat depression can occasionally cause confusion.

Severe depression can look like dementia in several ways.

Hypomania

Depressive illness is often a recurrent problem that comes back years after successful treatment. In a minority of sufferers the disorder sometimes returns, not as depression but as hypomania – a condition in which people become restless and over active. In this state the sufferer may be not only over talkative but also physically over active, interfering in other people's lives, unable to 'slow down' and sometimes unable to sleep. Ideas often rush in on the sufferer and this is reflected in speech which may be very pressurised and 'fly' from one subject to another. Often the sufferer is impatient and irritable with others, sometimes elated and sometimes, paradoxically depressed. Although hypomania should not be confused with dementia, it sometimes is. Like depressive illness, hypomania responds to medical treatment, though the sufferer will often have to come into hospital for a while for his or her own protection. People who suffer from recurrent attacks of hypomania and depression are given the diagnosis of manic-depressive illness.

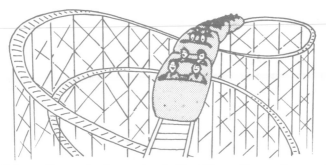

Living with manic-depression is like living with a rollercoaster mind.

Schizophrenia and paraphrenia

I have already mentioned that the dementia sufferer may accuse others of stealing mislaid property in an effort to make sense of the world. We often use the term 'paranoid' to describe this feeling of being persecuted by others. In the illness, schizophrenia, this idea is often much more definitely formed and elaborate. Memory is generally relatively well preserved but it may be impossible to test this because the sufferer will not cooperate or is 'in a world of his own'. Usually the patient will have suffered from the condition for some years and will be well known to the local psychiatric services. Sometimes, however, despite a long illness, the sufferer will only come to medical attention because a relative dies or some other stress of ageing leads to deterioration. Rarely, usually in isolated women who are often unmarried, a type of schizophrenia that occurs in older people, paraphrenia, may develop. None of these conditions should really be mistaken by a doctor for dementia, but they are mentioned here because they sometimes do look like 'confusion'. It is vital that they are not written off as dementia since, like depression and hypomania, they can be treated medically, usually with a remarkable degree of success.

47

Anxiety and other neuroses

In response to the stresses of old age, some people develop emotional disorders in which anxiety is the main characteristic (neuroses). Others have suffered from these problems all their lives, but they may get worse in old age. The symptoms of anxiety can take a number of forms. For example, the sufferer may experience palpitations, breathlessness, and 'butterflies' in the stomach. Sometimes the anxiety can be tied to specific situations and in this case it is called a phobia. The fear of going out (agoraphobia) is perhaps the best known of these fears. Unfortunately, although elderly people are not immune to them, agoraphobia and other neuroses are not noticed as often as they should be because of our lowered expectations of old people. Sometimes sufferers experience 'panic attacks' in certain situations. When this happens, anxiety suddenly builds up to such a pitch that the sufferer feels she or he has to escape. Often this panic is associated with overbreathing (hyperventilation), which upsets the biochemical balance of the body and can produce physical symptoms such as cramp and 'pins and needles' in the arm. The concentration of someone who is severely anxious can be so bad that they seem 'confused'. Again, this sort of problem should not be mistaken for dementia as it can often improve with medical or psychological treatment.

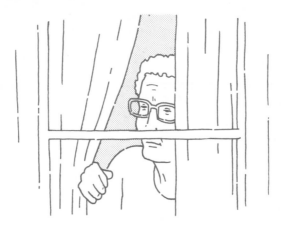

Many old people are afraid of going out.

Dysphasia

Sometimes a stroke can affect the part of the brain concerned with the understanding or expression of speech. Someone who has had a stroke may be unable to understand what other people say or to put words together to communicate with other people. This is called dysphasia and it is also a feature of various kinds of dementia. Rarely, however, a very small stroke can affect the speech area of the brain alone, leaving the victim physically and mentally otherwise intact. This is a very frightening experience for sufferers since when they hear other people it sounds like a 'foreign' language and when they try to speak, they may be quite unintelligible and distressed by their inability to make sense. This kind of condition can easily look like 'confusion' or 'dementia' but the facts that it comes on suddenly and the sufferer can still communicate by gesture and other non-verbal means should enable the distinction to be made. When someone suffers from dysphasia and multi-infarct dementia they may seem more confused than is really the case.

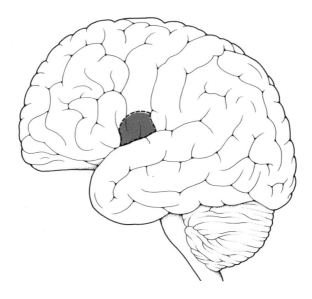

The area of the brain concerned with speech may be affected by a stroke.

Gerald was living in an old people's home when he was referred to Dr Wilkes, a psychiatrist, because of dementia, wandering, and disturbed behaviour. After seeing Gerald, Dr Wilkes was talking to a member of staff in the corridor (there being no office available), trying to explain that though he was demented, many of Gerald's problems stemmed from dysphasia, which made him seem more confused than he really was. This led staff to treat him as though he was severely demented, which in turn contributed to Gerald's disturbed behaviour. As Dr Wilkes was explaining this, Gerald 'wandered' past three times and on the third occasion managing to blurt out, 'You've left bag in my room doctor', demonstrating neatly the point that Dr Wilkes was making.

People with dysphasia can sometimes be helped by speech therapy and other people can assist too by speaking slowly, clearly, and simply. If questions are asked, they should only be asked one at a time and should permit a simple answer.

Alcohol and drugs

Alcohol and drugs can affect mental function but these are considered in detail on p. 53 and so will only be mentioned here.

7 Confusion—bodily causes

I explained earlier how various body systems change with age. Some of these changes are caused by ageing itself but others may be the result of repeated or longstanding illnesses. This means that the symptoms of an illness may be different from those seen in younger people. Doctors speak of 'non-specific presentations' of disease in old age. These are ways in which many different diseases can show themselves in the elderly, through problems such as repeated falls, immobility, and confusion.

Acute confusional states

The problem we are concerned with here, confusion caused by physical disorders, is called acute confusional state. It comes on suddenly and takes the form of restlessness, disorientation, memory problems, and a mood of perplexity or fear. Old people in an acute confusional state may misinterpret efforts to help and resist assistance or even become aggressive. They may sometimes see things that are not there, for example picking at imaginary insects on their clothes or bedclothes. This sort of confusion may be made worse by unsympathetic handling and a change of surroundings, as often happens when the sufferer is admitted to hospital.

The causes

Acute confusional states can be caused by illnesses in many different body systems but various infections (especially chest and urine infections) and heart failure are the most common.

51

Molly went to her GP, Dr Wells, complaining of breath-lessness. Dr Wells examined her and decided that she had a mild degree of heart failure which could be treated at home. Unfortunately, Molly suddenly became confused that evening and barricaded herself in her flat. She swore and threw things at neighbours who tried to get in to help her. Dr Wells was called and managed to calm her a bit. She decided that the acute confusional state was probably due to Molly's heart failure and arranged for her to be admitted to hospital. Molly's confusion went completely after her heart failure was brought under control.

Even small things can cause problems

In people who already have dementia, relatively small problems such as constipation can cause an increase in restlessness and confusion. If this is not recognised, the sufferer may remain needlessly uncomfortable and more confused than is necessary with the resultant extra burden on the carers.

Limiting the problem

Because the underlying causes of acute confusional states can often be treated, sufferers can be expected to recover to their previous mental state before the episode of acute confusion. In the meantime, a great deal can be done to limit the confusion. Someone they know should stay with the confused person whenever possible, especially if they have to go to hospital. Their room should be kept well lit and the sufferer gently and simply reminded what is happening. From the psychological point of view, the worst thing that can happen for an acutely confused old person is to be carried off to hospital by uniformed strangers (ambulancemen!) who then leave him or her to be seen by a series of nurses and doctors all of whom ask seemingly meaningless questions. Although confusion is inevitably worsened by going into hospital, the effect can be greatly lessened if a familiar person travels with the old person to explain (repeatedly if necessary) exactly what is happening, and if the hospital takes care to deal with the patient promptly, courteously, and with as few different staff as possible. possible.

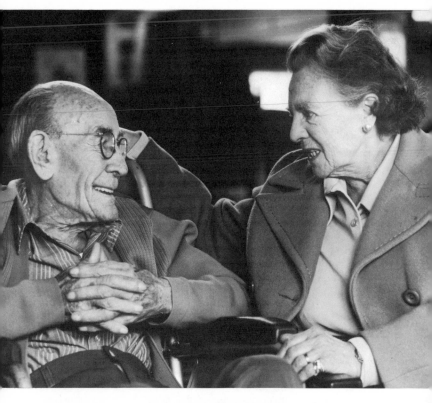

Confused old people take comfort from familiar faces

Drugs and alcohol

Although in the newspapers 'drugs' usually refers to drugs of abuse, the medical profession also uses the term to refer to all the medications used to treat people. Here, however, we are mainly, but not exclusively, concerned with 'psychotropic' drugs – drugs that act on the brain. Strictly speaking, alcohol, which people drink because it relaxes them and reduces social tensions and inhibitions, should be classed as a psychotropic drug.

53

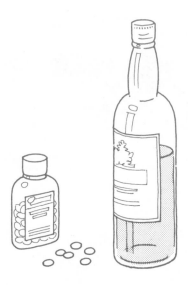

How drugs cause confusion

Drugs can cause confusion in a number of ways. Some cause confusion by acting longer than is necessary. For example, the sedative effect of sleeping tablets may last well into the day, causing a muddled feeling in the morning. Furthermore, some sleeping tablets may build up in the body over a period of days or weeks, leading to gradually increasing day time drowsiness and possible confusion.

Other drugs may have side effects that cause confusion. The brain's chemical messenger, acetylcholine, is involved in memory systems (see p.38) but certain drugs, notably some used to treat depression (antidepressants) anxiety, and paranoid symptoms (sedatives), affect this chemical messenger. They can produce confusion in mentally normal old people or worsen confusion in those who are already demented.

Drug interactions

Another problem may be interaction between different drugs. Alcohol can interact with most psychotropic drugs to cause drowsiness and confusion. Usually these drugs carry a warning on the packet that alcohol should be avoided but not everyone reads or remembers the warning! Whenever you have to call the doctor out, it is very important to tell him exactly what medications the patient is already taking, including those that have been bought over the chemist's counter.

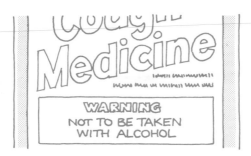

More about alcohol

- Alcohol is a sedative drug and drunkenness can be viewed as a self induced, acute confusional state.
- Long term over use of alcohol can result in dependence so that the sufferer actually needs the next drink. Without medical treatment, a dependent drinker who suddenly stops drinking alcohol may experience withdrawal symptoms which over a few hours or days, can develop into a severe, acute confusional state – delerium tremens or 'the DTs'. This can be a life threatening condition.
- Long term excessive drinking can cause liver damage that in turn may hasten confusion or even coma.
- Excessive drinking can produce brain damage and dementia by the direct, poisonous effect of alcohol on the brain or through vitamin deficiencies (especially thiamine deficiency) that occur in alcoholics who eat poorly.
- Finally, excessive drinking may contribute to raised blood pressure, one of the 'risk factors' for multi-infarct dementia (see chapter 5).

Tobacco

Smoking is generally bad for health. Tobacco, by contributing to heart and circulatory diseases, may also increase the risk of multi-infarct dementia.

8 Confusion—the senses and surroundings

Hearing

Our senses and environment will be considered together because they are so closely linked. Old age often brings with it some deterioration in hearing and vision. Hearing loss may be caused by the ageing of the systems connected with the ear or by exposure to loud noise over many years. It may also be simply due to wax in the ears, which can be treated by special ear drops or syringing. For other forms of hearing loss a hearing aid is often helpful. Old people are often embarrassed about wearing these and those who already have dementia may find it hard to adapt but it is generally worth persevering – a number of 'confused' old people turn out to be much less confused when they can hear what is going on!

Sight

Sight, too, may deteriorate because of ageing or because of age related disease, but many sight problems caused by getting older can be corrected by appropriate spectacles. Cataracts become increasingly common in old age. In this condition, the front part of the eye, the len, is unable to transmit light properly. Someone with cataracts who is already confused and is perhaps rushed to hospital because of another illness is going to find it particularly hard to interpret what is going on because they cannot see. Cataracts can be removed surgically when they are fully developed and a replacement lens can be fitted to the eye, or special spectacles may be provided after operation.

Spectacles and aids need checking

Spectacles and hearing aids can become useless for a variety of reasons.

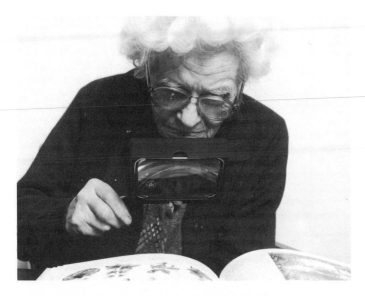

The spectacles may have been purchased many years ago and may no longer be suitable for the wearer. They may, especially if someone is suffering from dementia, be allowed to get excessively dirty. They may be lost and never replaced. Hearing aid batteries run flat and wax can block the ear mould. Sometimes the devices can simply break down. Most old people take care of these things for themselves but if there is a degree of confusion from other causes they may need help.

Prepare old people for changes

We have already stressed the importance of managing change in the surroundings for old people who are physically ill or suffering from an acute confusional state. This is equally important if someone suffering from dementia needs to go into hospital or a residential home.

Time and care is needed to prepare confused old people for these changes as far as they are able to understand them. Confusion may be worse for a time after any change in surroundings. This must be expected and coped with by skilled

57

and familiar staff. Friends and relatives may be enlisted to sit with the old person and explain what is happening. With patient teaching and as they begin to settle, confused residents can sometimes learn the way around, including the way to the toilet. The use of name plates on doors and familiar personal furnishings in their room can help too. Colour coding and even signposting of toilets in public areas will assist many, more mildly confused people to find their way about. Trained staff who can give the old people stimulating things to do and some physical exercise during the day can improve night time sleep. The same principles can be used at home for confused old people who do not need residential care.

Confusion may be worse for a time after any change in surroundings.

Prompts can help

Relatives can leave notes to remind those living alone to lock the door or only to cook for one. For many less confused people, the telephone can be used in a similar way to prompt the sufferer to remember important activities, for example to get up in the morning and be ready for the transport to the day centre. Behind all these ideas (and many more thought up by ingenious relatives) is the principle that people with some memory impairment can respond to 'cues' in the environment. In the same way that spectacles and hearing aids can be used to correct for poor vision and hearing, so these prompts can, in a limited way, correct for poor memory.

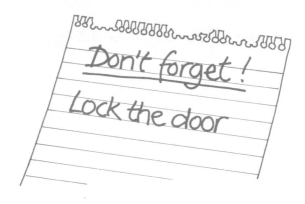

9 More about drugs

There is as yet no effective medical treatment for most cases of dementia in old age. Very occasionally dementia is caused by an underlying vitamin B12 deficiency. This can be identified by a simple blood test and can be treated with regular injections of vitamin B12, which have to be continued for life. Often, over a period of months, the sufferer's mental state will improve though they are not always completely restored to their previous ability. Deficiency of the thyroid hormone, thyroxine, is another rare and potentially treatable cause of dementia. In this case treatment is by tablets and again improvements may be seen over weeks and months. There are other, even rarer, causes of dementia for which surgical treatment can help.

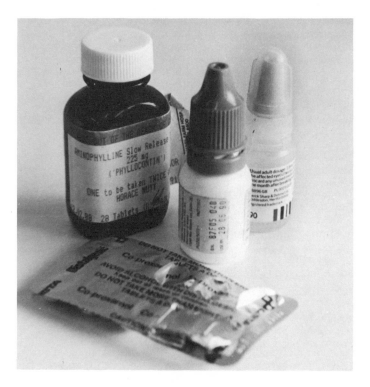

No really effective treatments

For the vast majority of old people with Alzheimer's disease and multi-infarct dementia, however, there are, as yet, no really effective medical treatments. There are a number of drugs that are supposed to increase the blood supply to the brain or the efficiency with which it works but none are of sufficient value to be routinely recommended. As mentioned earlier, in multi-infarct dementia, low doses of aspirin (perhaps as little as half a tablet every other day) may reduce, though not eliminate, the risk of further episodes of deterioration. As it is the cholinergic system (the mechanism by which nerve messages are sent through the brain) that is affected in Alzheimer's disease (see p.38) attempts have been made to improve dementia by giving sufferers choline or lecithin, both substances which the body can convert into the neurotransmitter, acetylocholine. Unfortunately, these attemps have not produced results sufficiently encouraging to justify everyday use. Other medications are currently being evaluated which mimic the effect of acetyl-choline in the brain but so far none have been proved to have a major effect on the course of Alzheimer's disease.

Drugs that control behaviour

Most medications prescribed in dementia are used to control particular problems rather than to treat the disease. This is perhaps broadly similar to the use of drugs for pain relief. Drugs that relieve pain do not usually cure the underlying illness but they are nevertheless worthwhile.

The control of disturbing behaviour in dementia is likewise worthwhile but two important reservations have to be made. Firstly, the medication is often being given not for the direct benefit of the patient but for the benefit of the carers. Secondly, side effects may sometimes outweigh benefit, particularly when drugs are prescribed for a long time.

Risks v benefits

Several groups of drugs used for the psychiatric treatment of confused old people will be briefly discussed here. In each case a few examples of the drugs within each group will be given. This is a short account intended to alert you to the potential benefits and drawbacks of medication. Prescribing medication in an individual case is very much a question of balancing risks against benefits. If you have any worries about particular medications please discuss them with your family doctor.

Tranquillisers and sleeping tablets

Most sleeping tablets and tranquillisers belong to a group of drugs called the benzodiazepenes, which includes nitrazepam (Mogadon), diazepam (Valium), chlordiazepoxide (Librium), lorazepam (Ativan) and many others. Those drugs produce a feeling of calmness and in higher doses induce sleep. They are remarkably safe if too many are taken. Many of these drugs, however, accumulate over weeks or months in old people if taken regularly and they can interfere with memory, cause excessive drowsiness, lead to falls, and be habit forming. Furthermore, if they are stopped suddenly after long term use there may be a rebound of anxiety or sleeplessness. For sleeplessness, other measures should always be tried first (see p.64) Although some old people have been on long term treatment with these drugs for years without serious adverse effects, others have suffered memory and other problems and most doctors now agree that they should be used sparingly and then, generally, only for a matter of a few days or weeks.

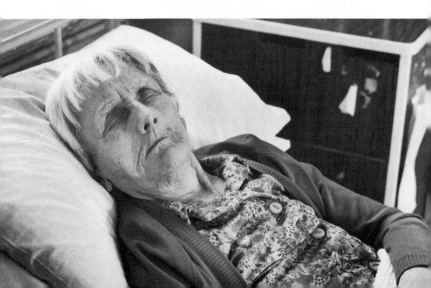

Major tranquillisers

Another, different group of tranquillisers were initially developed for the treatment of schizophrenia and related conditions. These are known as 'neuroleptics' or 'major tranquillisers' and include chlorpromazine (Largactil), haloperidol (Haldol), thioridazine (Melleril), and promazine (Sparine).

Drugs from this group are sometimes used to treat restlessness and other behaviour problems in patients with dementia. Major tranquillisers induce a feeling of calmness and to some extent control distressing hallucinations and false beliefs (found not only in schizophrenia but also to a lesser extent in dementia). Unfortunately they have a number of unwanted effects. They may produce slowness and rigidity in bodily movements. They may also have the opposite effect of causing restlessness and involuntary movements. Again, the best advice is to restrict their use in dementia as far as possible, though nobody would deny that they can sometimes be extremely helpful. The first step should always be to question whether there are alternative ways of dealing with problems (see p.88). If they must be used then they should be used in the smallest effective dose for a restricted period of time.

Antidepressants

These medications often affect the way nerve messages are sent and so can make confusion worse. Nevertheless, severe depression can co-exist with dementia, particularly in the early stages and in multi-infarct dementia, and cautious use of antidepressants can sometimes be useful. They will not be discussed in any detail here, however, since they are not primarily used for dementia. The main group is known as the tricyclic group of antidepressants because of their chemical structure. They include dothiepin (Prothiaden), amitriptyline (Tryptizol) and lofepramine (Gamanil). They can all cause dry mouth, constipation, and increased confusion, though lofepramine may cause fewer of these problems. Mianserin (Bolvidon) and fluvoxamine (Faverin) are more recent antidepressants with a different chemical structure and they have their own advantages and disadvantages.

Taking the drugs

When confused old people live alone it is often virtually impossible to ensure that they take their medicine properly. If they live with you, you should be alert to possible problems caused by drugs and should never be afraid to draw the doctor's attention to these.

Guidelines on medicines

Though this account has concentrated on possible problems associated with the use of medication in dementia, it must again be emphasised that drug treatment can sometimes be extremely helpful. The important principles are not to use medication if other measures can be found which are equally effective, to keep the dose and length of treatment to a minimum, and to report any possible drug induced problems to the doctor.

Other substances

Finally, it must be remembered that not all drugs are prescribed by doctors. Alcohol is technically a sedative drug and can interact with medication. A number of drugs can also be bought over the chemist's counter and these can sometimes produce adverse effects or have unwanted interactions with prescribed drugs. If in doubt ask your family doctor or the chemist for advice.

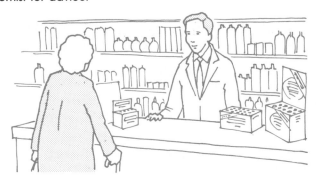

10 Problem behaviour

People with dementia and their relatives face many special problems. Not least among these are difficulties caused by other people's ignorance about dementia. One way in which this ignorance shows itself is in a tendency to over simplify the disorder by applying a label. Thus a sufferer is dismissed as 'senile', with the implication that 'nothing can be done'. Not only are these labels given to the sufferer, however, they are also used to cover whole classes of behaviour. 'Oh, he's violent' or 'she's a wanderer' may be useful shorthand but they say nothing of the circumstances in which violence or wandering may occur. They attribute the behaviour entirely to the person and take no account of factors in the surroundings or the way that other people may contribute to the behaviour.

Coping with problem behaviour

In this chapter, we are going to consider some areas of problem behaviour and see how these can be modified by the surroundings or the action of other people. The problems that have been chosen, lack of sleep, wandering, and aggression often affect people with dementia and their carers. One of the other major problem behaviours, incontinence, has already been discussed briefly on p.35 but will be considered in more detail here.

Lack of sleep

Perhaps more than anything else, the burden of not being able to get a good night's sleep can exhaust carers. The temptation for the doctor is to deal with this by prescribing sleeping pills for the sufferer, but although this may be justified in the short term, it is rarely effective in the long term and there may be a price to pay in increased drowsiness and confusion by day. As the chart shows there are a number of things that should be considered before a sleeping tablet is asked for (or prescribed).

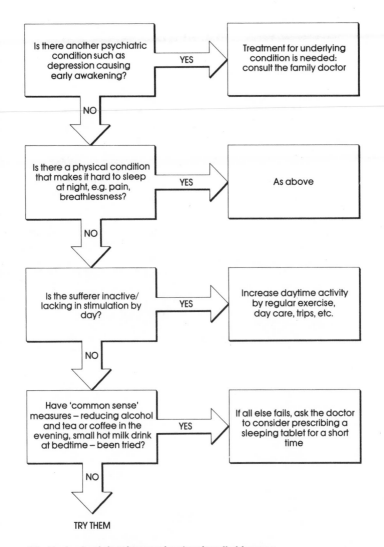

| Is there another psychiatric condition such as depression causing early awakening? | YES → | Treatment for underlying condition is needed: consult the family doctor |

NO ↓

| Is there a physical condition that makes it hard to sleep at night, e.g. pain, breathlessness? | YES → | As above |

NO ↓

| Is the sufferer inactive/ lacking in stimulation by day? | YES → | Increase daytime activity by regular exercise, day care, trips, etc. |

NO ↓

| Have 'common sense' measures – reducing alcohol and tea or coffee in the evening, small hot milk drink at bedtime – been tried? | YES → | If all else fails, ask the doctor to consider prescribing a sleeping tablet for a short time |

NO ↓

TRY THEM

What to do about sleeplessness in a 'confused' old person.

As with all behavioural problems, the successful solution does not lie in the label 'sleeplessness' but in looking behind the label for underlying problems to see if there are any that can be remedied.

65

Wandering

The first step in understanding this problem is to define what is meant. After all, 'wandering' can take many forms. A group of old ladies with dementia on a psychiatric ward used to go for a regular afternoon 'wander'. They would go out of the door, round the unit, and return. Although they needed to be watched in case they got lost, nine times out of 10 they would return without incident. There would have been no point in trying to stop this wandering – it had social value and provided necessary exercise.

Restlessness

In day care centres and residential homes it is very common for old people who are demented to become restless at tea time. In day care centres this restlessness may often start earlier, just after lunch and may be based on anxiety as to whether transport home will arrive. In residential care it may be related more often to a vague feeling that it is the end of the day and the sufferer should be 'going home'. In both situations, distraction will often work. Someone who is busy reminiscing about the past or joining in 'old time' singing is less likely to be anxious about 'getting out'.

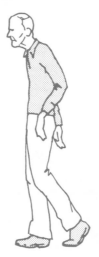

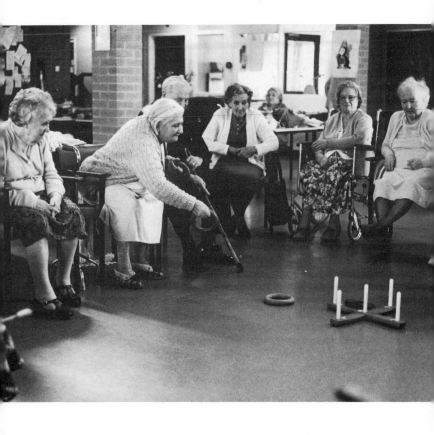

Locked door

Sometimes, however, the only thing that helps is a door with a double handle, combination lock, or other device to make it hard for the confused person to get out. Such a door is effectively 'locked' so far as the confused person is concerned but it should only be used in addition to techniques such as distraction, not as a substitute for them. Just as factors in the environment can help, they can also hinder. In day care centres, the practice of putting everyone's coat on before transport arrives is likely to increase restlessness and if several different vehicles arrive with a long interval between, the last people to leave are likely to be quite anxious by the time their transport arrives.

67

There may be underlying causes

'Wandering' may represent restlessness. When any old person with dementia develops increased restlessness, underlying causes should be sought – they may simply want to go to the toilet or perhaps the restlessness is caused by medication. Some sedative drugs can cause restlessness which shows itself in inability to remain in a seat. If this cause is not recognised, the amount of sedative may be increased in order to treat the symptom it is responsible for causing! Constipation is another common cause of restlessness in confused old people.

Insecurity

The temporary absence of a close carer may lead to apparently aimless searching. The demented person may not be able to remember that the carer has only gone into the kitchen to make tea and may follow them everywhere to keep them 'in sight'. Sometimes distraction will work. Sometimes the sufferer can be reassured simply by the voice of the carer, so that talking (or singing!) from the other room may be enough to prevent the searching starting. After bereavement, demented people can be particularly upset and restless. They may not be able to explain this or apparently even remember who has died but they may feel distressed and may go off searching for the lost one.

Violence is the voice of the unheard

Aggression

Once, as I was leaving a home where I had diagnosed dementia in the husband and explained to the wife something about the diagnosis, its implications, and the help we could offer, she took me on one side and asked 'do they get violent?' I was able to reassure her that violence is not normally part of the picture of dementia. Nevertheless, it does sometimes occur, and like other behavioural problems it has to be understood on an individual basis. Martin Luther King once said in a political context, 'Violence is the voice of the unheard' and this remark holds true for people with mental illness too.

Look behind aggression

Though the behaviour of someone with dementia may not make much sense to other people, from the point of view of the sufferer it is generally purposeful. The old lady may believe she has to get home to make tea for her children, the man that he has to go to work. When others try to restrain them they may become violent because of their 'unheard' need. This may be consistent with previous personality or may represent a loss of normal emotional control due to the dementia. This loss of emotional control is particularly common in patients with multi-infarct dementia in whom areas near the front of the brain concerned with the regulation of emotion have been damaged. Violence is usually provoked by confrontation, and confrontation often follows when an old person with dementia is trying to do something which is potentially unsafe.

> **Mr Howard was over 80. He had been demented for some years and lived with his devoted wife. He would get up in the middle of the night and, without getting dressed properly, would insist he must go to work. If his wife tried to stop him, he would hit out. She was much smaller than he and not very quick on her feet. She was trapped between allowing him to go out when she knew it was unsafe and putting herself in danger of being hit. Nor would the strategy of locking the door and hiding the key work. He would simply demand the key from her, and if she refused he might again become violent. She wanted to look after him as long as she could but eventually it became too much for her and he had to come into hospital. At first he proved very difficult to contain in hospital but then his physical condition deteriorated and he became easier to manage.**

Medication

Medication can sometimes help reduce violent outbursts. Strong (major) tranquillisers can make an aggressive person more docile but there are often side effects of this drug treatment such as stiffness, restlessness, and tremor. Some other drugs such as one used for treating epilepsy, carbamazepine, and the mood controlling drug, lithium, can sometimes have an effect in controlling violence but they also have side effects and risks and do not always work, even if the sufferer can be persuaded to take them. Obviously the use of these drugs is a matter for the family doctor, in consultation with the specialist when necessary.

Fear causes aggression

Sometimes aggression may simply result from fear on the part of a sufferer who does not know what is going on.

One lady, Joan, in her mid 90s was living with her daughter. She had gradually become demented and at the same time had become blind and deaf in ways that could not be treated. Joan became aggressive whenever anyone tried to dress, undress, or wash her. Clearly she did not know what was going on. Nor did she know what time of the day it was as she was unable to see whether it was light or dark. A combination of night time restlessness and daytime violence was endured by her daughter for some time. Fortunately, Joan would still go to the day care centre and this at least provided some respite. When Joan started to refuse this too, however, her daughter could no longer cope and admission to hospital, followed by transfer to residential care was organised. Staff noted that Joan was a pleasant old lady who simply did not like being disturbed. Because she could not see or hear the staff were unable to follow their usual practice of telling her when they were going to wash or dress her but noted that although she sometimes fought when they started to do these things, once she had realised what they were trying to do, she would 'settle down' and even stroke them as if in compensation for her earlier violence.

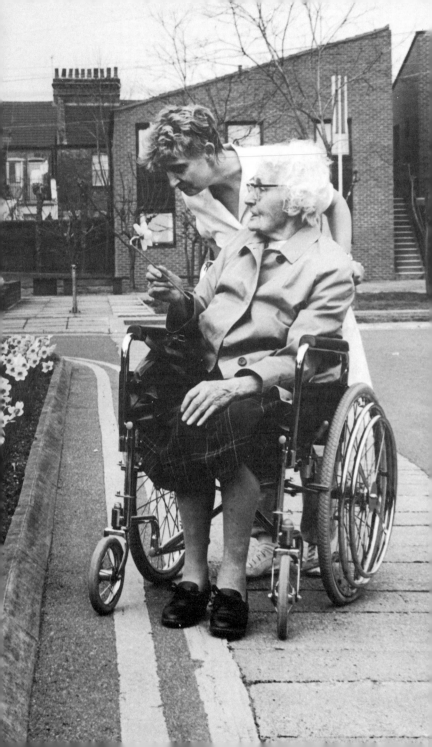

Incontinence

This subject has already been mentioned on p.35. Like many 'problem' behaviours it can have many different causes. Incontinence is rarely due to dementia itself, although in the very late stages of the disease, the capacity to control the passing of urine and of stools may be lost. Few people live long enough, however, to develop dementia so severe as to produce this type of incontinence. More commonly the cause for incontinence is physical.

Poor mobility

One of the most important factors in incontinence is poor mobility, which in turn may be due to other problems, for example arthritis, that can sometimes be treated medically. Mobility is also relative. Toilets which are too far away from day areas or bedrooms can make it impossible for some old people to reach them in time.

Other physical causes

Another physical cause is a urinary infection, which is common in old people but can be treated with antibiotics. And remember that poor sight can lead to the sufferer being unable to find the toilet without help.

Mrs Smith suffered from diabetes and was also totally blind. Her husband cared for her at home but when his health broke down, she had to go into residential care. Although staff initially described her as 'very confused', when she was assessed it was obvious that she had some grasp of what was happening. Staff at the home were not used to dealing with blind people but they responded quickly to her daytime calls for the toilet and led her there. At night though she was often incontinent and staff thought this was probably because of the layout and night staffing levels of the home which meant that her night time calls for help in finding the toilet were not responded to as quickly as they would have liked.

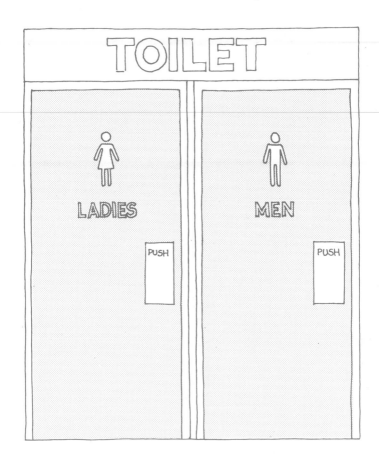

Toilets should be easily seen

Not only may toilets be too far away, they may also be too hard to recognise or get into. Some hospital wards have sliding toilet doors which demented old people may find hard to operate. Ideally, toilet doors should be easy to open, well labelled and, in hospital or residential care, be well signposted and painted in a bright consistent colour different from that of any other doors. In this way it will be easier for sufferers' to find the toilet unaided and the risks of incontinence will be reduced.

Attention-seeking behaviour

I have already mentioned that other people may sometimes inadvertently encourage incontinence and other problem behaviour by paying attention only when the unwanted behaviour happens. If such a pattern of behaviour starts to emerge, it is worth looking at what is happening immediately beforehand, what the behaviour itself is, and what the consequences of the behaviour are. If a demented old person who wants attention learns that they get this *only* when they are doing something that carers do not like, they will be encour-

How Mrs J's incontinence was 'encouraged'

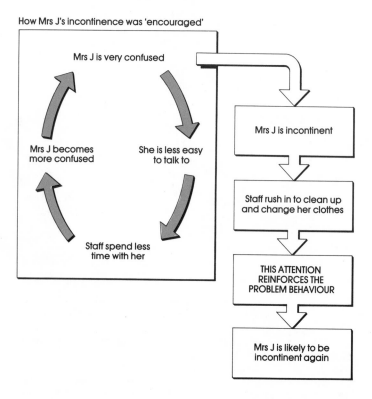

Mrs J's incontinence.

aged into problem behaviour. This phenomenon is known as 'reinforcement' and the diagram illustrates how it may occur.

Once the problem has been recognised, then plans can be made to reduce the reinforcement of the unwanted behaviour and, even more important, to encourage other wanted behaviour (for example, by involving the resident in pleasurable conversation and reminiscence, or at least by sitting with them, when they are not 'misbehaving').

Behavioural management

When a behaviour problem occurs people often give it a 'label' and then accept it, as though they believe that naming the problem is the most that can be expected. In fact, by systematically working through the possible causes in the brain, the body, the senses (especially hearing and vision), and the surroundings, some problems can be reduced or even eliminated. Simple psychological principles, such as reinforcement, drawn from the study of human behaviour allow us to change people's behaviour indirectly by changing our response to it. Of course, expert help may be needed in applying these principles but I mention them here because they are so important and because they can often be of great practical use.

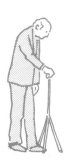

11 The helping services

The services needed by dementia sufferers and their relatives are currently provided by several groups – health authorities, local authorities, voluntary agencies, and the private sector. Despite, or perhaps partly because of, the multitude of different sources of help, some vital services·are not available in some places or don't have enough resources. A review of care currently available in the community was recently undertaken on behalf of the Department of Health and Social Security (DHSS) by Sir Roy Griffiths, and this may well lead to a more even distribution of services. It is, however, unlikely to lead to a much needed injection of money. Indeed, some people fear that by bringing in strict government controls over expenditure on voluntary and private residential and nursing homes a current 'safety valve' may be lost. At present, the money available for local authority residential homes has failed to keep pace with the expansion of the very elderly population. At the same time, the private sector, largely financed through public money (in the form of various DHSS benefits paid to residents), has expanded to fill the gap. If this development now comes under tight central control, it seems likely that already inadequate resources will be stretched to breaking point. In the section that follows, the provision of services by each of the groups mentioned above will be considered in turn.

> **Services for dementia sufferers are provided by • health authorities, • local authorities, • voluntary agencies, • and the private sector.**

Local health district provision

The family doctor service is provided through local health authorities. Family doctors are often the first contact for carers worried about confusion in a relative and they can do a great deal in making a medical diagnosis of the underlying cause. If there is a treatable cause for the confusion, for example a

76

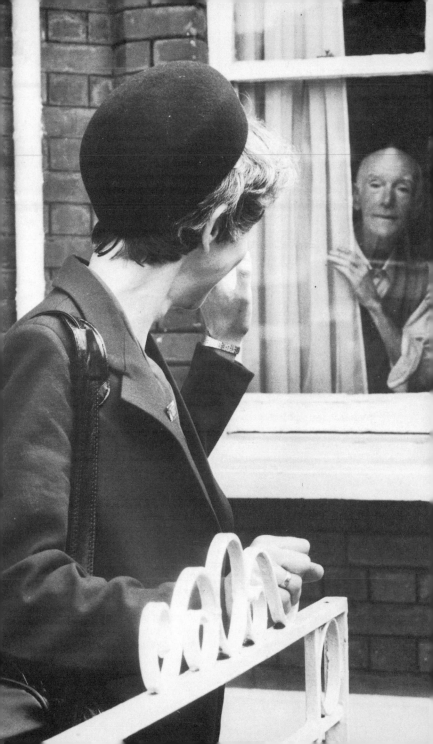

physical illness causing an acute confusional state, depressive illness causing 'pseudo-dementia', or a reversible vitamin deficiency, family doctors can start treatment and call on expert help from specialists if needed.

The family doctor can also advise the family about getting help from social services when appropriate. In addition, where rehousing, residential, or nursing home care is needed he or she may be able to argue the case with the authorities for a 'medical' priority to be given to the patient. Family doctors are often uniquely placed to understand the family stresses and strains caused by an ill member. Their ability to respond to these problems will depend, however, on their training and on how much time is available. Generally speaking, doctors working in inner city areas are more hard pressed because of the greater number of medical and social problems among their patients.

The district nurse

The district nurse works with the family doctor in the primary care team and can provide a limited amount of nursing supervision in the patient's home. He or she can, for example, help deal with constipation and other physical problems. They can also, to a limited extent, help supervise medication. They do not generally have special training in dealing with elderly confused people but nevertheless they can often provide important support.

When incontinence occurs, despite all attempts to cure it, district nurses are often the agency through whom specialised incontinence garments and other aids can be supplied. In some health distrcts district nurses are backed up by specially trained nurses whose role is to advise on the maintenance of continence and the provision of aids when necessary.

Health visitor and community nurse

Although health visitors have a primarily preventive role and have traditionally concentrated on child care, a small number are now beginning to take an interest in preventive care of old people. Some family doctors also have direct access to community psychiatric nurses whose role is to provide expert nursing assessment and care (including the coordination of other appropriate services). As they are mainly based in hospital teams, however, community psychiatric nurses will be discussed later.

Medical specialists

In addition to referring patients for nursing help, family doctors can refer old people for home assessment by a hospital based physician or psychiatrist, often a specialist in the physical or mental problems of old people. In some health districts, the family doctor may also be able to refer his patient to a psychologist for special help. Unlike psychiatrists, psychologists do not have a medical training and cannot prescribe drugs. They have a very detailed training in the science of human behaviour, however, and can offer a wide range of help based on this training. Like community psychiatric nurses, psychologists often work as part of a team of specialists based in hospital. There are a whole range of other people from chiropodists to opticians to whom family doctors can turn for help in dealing with some of the important associated problems of confused old people.

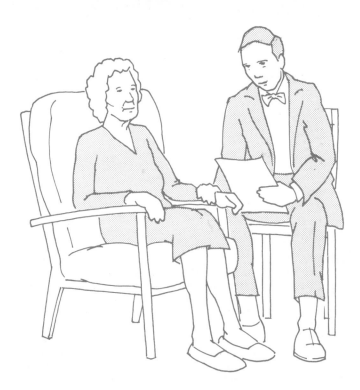

The family doctor is important

Family doctors have a very wide role in diagnosing and, where possible treating the underlying causes of confusion. They are uniquely placed to understand the impact of dementia on relatives and they can call in specialist help when required. Unfortunately, prescribing medicines is sometimes seen as the family doctor's only role, and occasionally tablets are prescribed that make matters worse. If this happens it is very important to draw the doctor's attention to the problems. It is equally important that when a doctor (who may be a locum) calls out of hours and does not know the patient that relatives can explain exactly what medication is being taken, especially as the locum doctor may not have access to the patient's medical records.

Hospital services

The main hospital services involved in the care of demented old people are psychiatric and geriatric medical services. In the event of an urgent illness, however, almost any department of the hospital may be called upon. For example, a demented old person who breaks a leg will be referred to the orthopaedic department. When this happens, it is vitally important that the special needs of the demented patient are recognised and met.

Specialised psychiatric services

About 70% of the elderly population in Britain now have a specialised psychiatric service for old people available to them, and the proportion covered is increasing all the time. Specialised consultants will usually work in a team with other doctors, community nurses, occupational therapists, and perhaps a clinical psychologist and a physiotherapist. They can generally call on a small specialised day hospital unit and ward for those who need inpatient treatment. In addition they are 'gate-keepers' for admission of severely demented patients to long-stay hospital facilities. When called in, the psychiatrist or one of the team will usually make an initial assessment of the sufferer at home. Usually the services of the specialist team are called in by the family doctor but sometimes the social worker does this with the family doctor's consent. A few services take referrals directly form the family but all prefer to work with the knowledge and consent of the family doctor.

After the patient has been assessed

After the initial assessment, the specialist may ask the patient to attend an outpatients clinic, or the day hospital, or even to come into the ward for a brief period of assessment. The specialist may also bring in other members of the team who can provide support for the old person at home or recommend a course of action to the local social services department. The family, if available, will generally be an important source of information for the specialist assessment and they will usually be involved in plans for future assessment, treatment, and care of the sufferer.

The community psychiatric nurse

The community psychiatric nurse often has an important role in seeing patients at home on a regular basis to check on how well they are, to provide or supervise treatment, and to help with many other problems. If an old person fails to attend hospital when they should it is often the community nurse who is called out to see what is happening.

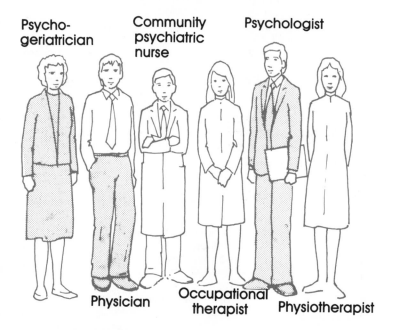

Psycho-geriatrician

Community psychiatric nurse

Psychologist

Physician

Occupational therapist

Physiotherapist

Physical problems

If the patient's main problem at the time of referral is thought to be a physical illness, the family doctor will generally call in the local specialist physician in geriatric medicine. He or she may admit the patient to hospital or may see the patient at home or in the outpatient clinic.

Social services

Local social services authorities are responsible for providing a range of support to old people in their own homes. Regular hot meals, laundry service, home helps, and daily wardens are amongst the most important services for confused old people. For some, regular attendance at a day centre can provide a focus for the week or much needed relief for families. Local authorities also provide residential care for old people who need it. This may be on an occasional basis to provide a break for families or it may be long term. Other schemes such as family placement (where the old person is cared for by a carefully selected family) and 'sitting' services (where someone comes in to give the carer a well deserved break) are sometimes available.

If you want to get in touch with your local social services department look up the number in the telephone directory and discuss any help needed with them. If a specific service is requested, such as a home help, there will generally be some form of assessment to see exactly what is required. If more general help is asked for, a social worker or social welfare officer may make the assessment. These workers may also offer emotional support to carers.

Social services provide

- Regular hot meals;
- Laundry service;
- Home helps;
- Daily wardens;
- Day centres;
- Residential care.

Private agencies

Encouraged by government policies, the private sector has recently developed rapidly in offering residential and nursing home care to old people. In some areas, especially in the South of England, this development has been so great that the local geriatric and psychiatric services and even social services have been able to reduce their own provision. Generally speaking, the residents in private homes are less disabled than those found in local authority residential care, who correspond more closely in disability to patients in private nursing homes.

Planning is a problem

Since private developments are largely independent, it is hard for health and social service authorities to include them in overall plans. In some cities, the large houses around the old parks are being converted into private residential and nursing homes at an alarming rate. This can have the effect of concentrating disabled old people in particular areas which causes increased and unexpected demand on local health services. Because there is no central planning of these private developments some areas of the country are relatively richly provided with private care whereas others have very little. We hope that one of the benefits of the Griffiths review of community care will be a more integrated approach to planning and provision of services.

Private community services

Although private social work, home help, and other community services are developing, the emphasis in the private sector has, so far been on residential facilities and this has therefore been the area of most rapid development in recent years. Community services have simply not kept pace with the changing age structure of the population.

Voluntary agencies

In some countries, voluntary and church groups have been responsible for extensive provision and new ideas in the care of old people. The housing associations in this country have done a great deal towards providing sheltered housing but voluntary groups have not so far made the impact on residential and nursing home care that they have made in some other countries. There has, however, been notable work by the Alzheimer's Disease Society, Age Concern, the Association of Carers, and other agencies in providing relatives support groups, telephone counselling services, home support, day care, and even pilot schemes for residential care for confused old people. A list of potentially helpful organisations is provided on p.101.

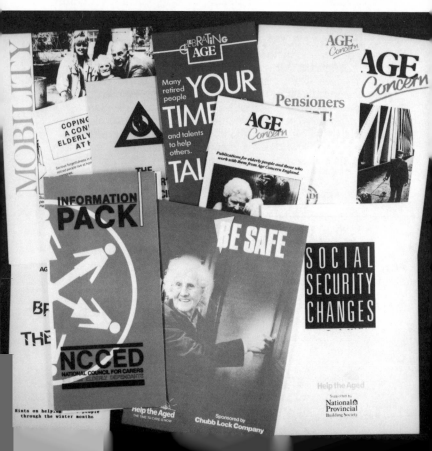

Residential and nursing home care

Dementia sufferers are often unable to make rational choices for themselves but they should always be involved in making decisions about their own care when practicable. Unfortunately, shortage of resources in local authority services often means that little or no choice can be offered. In the private sector there is much more choice in some areas than others. Dementia sufferers may, however, be seen as 'problem patients' and may be excluded from many residential homes. When demented people are being cared for at public expense, whether in the public or private sectors, there is little financial allowance made for their high supervision needs. In these circumstances, relatives, friends, and other caregivers should assess the quality of care being provided and complain to the authorities if necessary.

Principles of care for dementia sufferers

The care of dementia sufferers should be founded on the fact that they have basically the same rights and needs as other people. At the same time their individuality should be respected and their special needs provided for. It is simply not acceptable to have large communal dormitory areas, toilet facilities which lack privacy, and no space for personal provisions. Guidelines have been provided for residential care in documents such as *Home Life* (see book list, on p.102) but here a few points are stressed to assist relatives in assessing the residential care provided, whether by the NHS, the local authority, a voluntary agency, or privately:

Assessing residential care

- Does the home offer adequate privacy?
- Are staff sufficient in number and training to provide adequate care?
- Are there plenty of daytime activities for those who want them?
- Are the residents allowed the maximum choice they are capable of exercising in terms of daily time schedule, etc?
- Is the general atmosphere pleasant and friendly or rigid and authoritarian?
- Are residents treated as individuals?

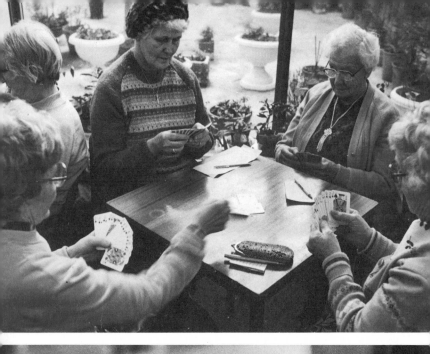

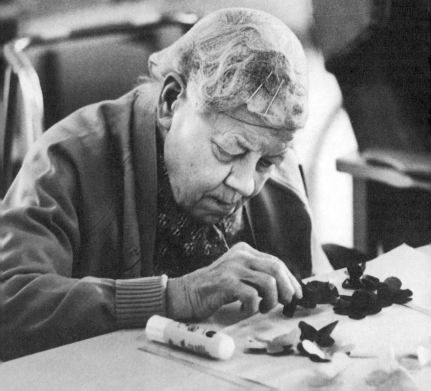

- Is there some security of tenure?
- How is disturbed behaviour dealt with? Is it tolerated inappropriately so that other residents suffer, is it rigidly suppressed by drug treatment or a requirement that the disturbed person go elsewhere, or is it coped with constructively with expert help from the psychiatric services if necessary?

Monitoring is currently inadequate

There are books which set out in much more detail the principles of good residential care (for example, *Living well into old age*, see p.102). Since many demented old people in these settings are unable to monitor the quality of their own care, it is particularly important for friends and relatives to do this for them. There are statutory inspections of health and social services facilities by the Health Advisory Service and of private residential and nursing home facilities by the local social services and health authorities. However, in the case of the former, recommendations are not necessarily needed and in the case of the latter the local authorities' only sanction is to close substandard homes, which leaves them with the problem of finding accommodation for displaced residents – hardly an incentive to rigorous inspection!

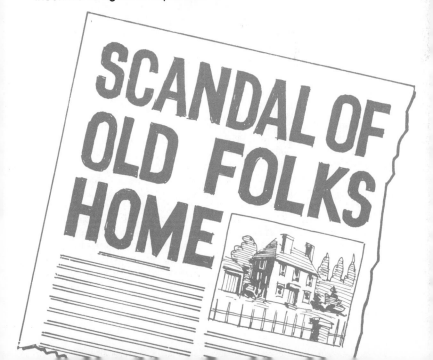

12 What can I do?

Nearly always, the person asking for help is the carer not the sufferer. Few problems engender a greater feeling of helplessness than seeing a loved one become confused, particularly if that confusion is believed to be caused by an irreversible dementia. Often, the first thing you have to cope with is that the sufferer does not recognise the problem and denies the need for any help. Yet help is essential for both of you.

Ask for an assessment

In practically every confused old person, an early medical assessment is useful. You may have to take the initiative in contacting the family doctor who will then see the patient at home or at the surgery, whichever is more appropriate. If necessary the family doctor can take blood tests or call in specialist help for further assessment. You may have to act as advocate for the sufferer in ensuring that appropriate help is received. You can also get in touch directly with the local social services department to arrange community services. In some areas telephone information and counselling services run by groups such as Alzheimer's Disease Society can help you find your way through the maze of helping agencies.

Carers need help too

If the first step for carers is to ask for appropriate help for sufferers, the second is to ask for appropriate help for themselves. This is not only with practical problems such as home support, day care, and legal questions but also for coping with the emotional problems of 'living bereavement'. Mutual support groups, organised by a variety of agencies, serve two purposes – they provide information and give emotional support to carers. A list of some of the voluntary agencies which may be involved in or know of local relative support groups is given later in chapter 13. Local social services offices and your family doctor may also be involved in, or know of, these groups. Sometimes, especially if it is your spouse or other close relative that is affected, you may suffer such a severe reaction and distress that you need antidepressant drugs, psychiatric help, or psychological counselling. Do be prepared for this possibility and seek help as soon as possible. Most specialised psychiatric services for old people consider the support of carers to be one of their primary duties.

Remember that many carers find the problems so distressing that they need expert medical help themselves.

You may need to be 'pushy'

As well as seeking assessment for sufferers, you need to act as their advocate in ensuring that the standard of help they receive is adequate. This may mean pestering already overworked professionals as well as monitoring the effects of any help (including medical treatments) to report back to the various agencies trying to help. These agencies should recognise your central role and involve you in planning care for long term dementia sufferers. If they don't do this, then you must campaign to be recognised.

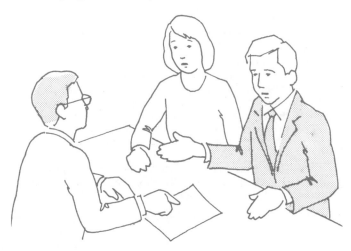

In situations where the professionals are unable to deliver adequate help, caregivers can complain to the local health authority, community health council or, in the case of social services, their local councillor. Dementia sufferers are themselves rarely able to complain constructively about services and this places an extra duty on doctors, nurses, social workers, other caring professionals, relatives, and friends.

Can anything be done to help a damaged memory?

The reality orientation approach to care of the dementia sufferer is extremely useful for caregivers. This approach tries to compensate for the sufferer's failing memory by giving as much information about what is going on as the sufferer can cope with. The sufferer's day is given some structure and cues are organised to remind him or her of what is going on. Used in a way that is sensitive to the specific abilities and needs of the sufferer, this approach can help reduce (though not 'cure') confusion and give you a rational way of planning help. An excellent book on this topic *Reality Orientation*, by Una Holden and Robert Woods is available (see chapter 13). As an example of the influence of reality orientation imagine the following two scenes.

Scenario 1
It is 8.30 in the morning. Mrs Brown who has been confused for about two years and lives alone is in bed. Someone knocks at the door. She struggles out of bed and gets down to the door, opening it to see who's there. It is a man in a dark uniform whom she takes to be a policeman. 'Are you ready then,' he says. 'What for, I didn't ask for you to come,' replies Mrs Brown.

'I've come to take you to the hospital.' 'What for, there's nothing wrong with me,' she answers and shuts the door in his face.

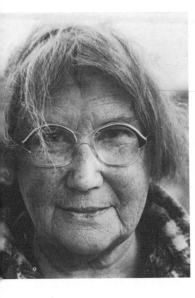

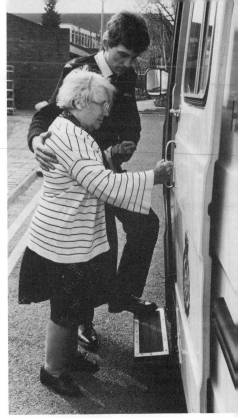

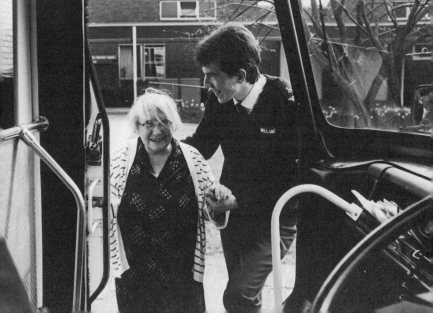

Scenario 2

It is 7.00 in the morning. The telephone by Mrs Brown's bed rings. It is the familiar voice of her daughter: 'Hello, mum. It's Tuesday morning. I'm phoning to remind you that today's your day to go to the day hospital. It's 7 o'clock now, so you'd better get up and get dressed ready for Betty who's coming to help you with breakfast.'

Half an hour later, the doorbell rings. Mrs Brown is already up, though still in her dressing gown. She recognises the face of the lady at the door though she can't remember who she is.

'Hello Mrs Brown, it's me, Betty; I always come to help you get ready to go out on Tuesday. Can I come in?'

By the time the ambulance arrives, Mrs Brown is dressed and fed. She has just been to the toilet. As the ambulance draws up outside, Betty says 'Here's the bus to take you to the day hospital – you'll be back at about 4 o'clock and I'll leave some sandwiches and a flask of tea to warm you up when you come in. Again the face at the door is a familiar one. Because she has been prepared for the driver, Mrs Brown is quite cooperative.

Reality orientation makes a difference

The same lady seems awkward and uncooperative in the first scene but friendly and pleased to cooperate in the second. She has not changed; but in the second scene, those around her are making proper allowance for her disability. Few of us would expect a blind person to cross a busy road unaided but it is amazing how often we expect someone with impaired memory to remember what is going on. Reality orientation is all about treating memory impairment like any other disability, and compensating for it.

Reminiscence

Another approach used often in day centres, day hospitals, and residential settings is reminiscence. This uses the strategy, also common in helping the physically handicapped, of making maximum use of residual abilities. Old people with dementia often enjoy talking about the past and are still good at relating to other people in groups. Reminiscence uses old photographs or familiar objects from the past to stimulate discussion on a one to one or group basis. Reminiscence can also help younger staff to appreciate the historical reality of the harsh times and the joys that old people have experienced as part of their personal histories. At the end of the session it is important not to leave the old people 'in the past' but to bring them back to present reality.

Make a scrapbook

Related to this approach is the practice of making a personal scrapbook of the sufferer's previous life, with old photographs, marriage announcements, long service certificates, and other personal memorabilia. Items should be carefully labelled and you can also paste in up to date photos of family and friends. This personal scrapbook can go with the old person if he or she has to go into hospital or residential care and can help care staff get to know the 'real person' locked inside by the memory loss of dementia.

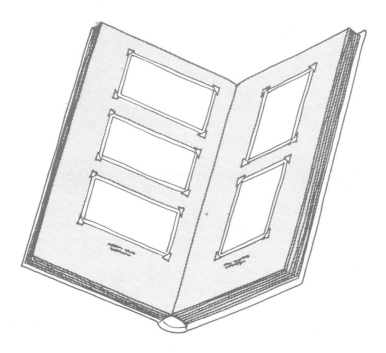

Where should the sufferer live?

As far as possible dementia sufferers should be cared for in their own home and neighbourhood. If they live with you, then you will be able to cope more easily if you can make arrangements for them to receive some day care and short periods in residential care to give you a break. You can also make use of support services in the community. If the sufferer lives alone there comes a point when friends, relatives, and the caring agencies can no longer manage without unacceptable risk. As community care services improve and become more efficient and flexible, it is likely that this point will come at a later stage of disability. Whenever it comes, however, the options are generally a move to live with other family members, sisters, brothers, or children or a move into residential, nursing home, or long stay hospital care.

Give it thought

You and your family need to think long and hard before taking in demented relatives. Your ability to cope will depend on practical things like the size of the house, the number and age of your children, and the other commitments on your time. It will also depend on emotional things like the quality of previous relationships. It is not a decision to be taken lightly and expert advice should be sought if you are in any doubt. Professor Elaine Murphy's excellent book, *Dementia and Mental Illness in the Old* (see chapter 13) explores some of the issue in more depth.

What about financial and legal problems?

Old people who are demented may forget to pay their bills or to collect their pensions. Often informal arrangements can be made for a friend, relative, home help or social worker to help with these matters. In the early stages of dementia it is now legally possible for the sufferer to make a more formal arrangement called an enduring power of attorney, which can be held by a friend or relative. If the person is no longer capable of making a decision to give a power of attorney (and this is a matter in which legal and medical advice is generally needed) and there are substantial assets to be managed, then you should apply to the Court of Protection, which protects the interests of mentally incapacitated people. Generally, it is best to take expert advice from a solicitor on these matters, but local citizens advice bureaux may be able to help with general advice.

Financial help

Financial assistance may be available from the state, but as benefits are currently being reviewed it is essential to get up to date information. The local post office can usually provide explanatory leaflets and the citizens advice bureaux provide specialist advice. At present *supplementary pensions* are available for those on very low income. A person who is severely disabled (and this includes dementia) may be eligible for *attendance allowance* if their disability leads them to need attendance by day or night, or both. The allowance is paid to the sufferer so that he or she can 'buy in' needed services, but in practice for patients with dementia it can be used to help compensate caring relatives for loss of income from other sources as well as to purchase professional assistance. An *invalid care allowance* can be paid to a person below retirement age who spends a lot of time (over 35 hours per week) looking after someone in receipt of an attendance allowance. Sadly, *mobility allowance* is *not* usually available to old people – presumably they are not seen as needing to move around!

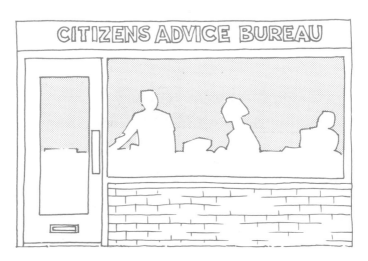

> The state benefits currently available include
> • supplementary pension, • attendance allowance,
> • invalid care allowance. These are being reviewed,
> however, so do get up to date information from your
> post office or citizens advice bureau.

The finances of residential care

When old people go into local authority residential care they are expected to contribute to their upkeep according to their means. In private residential and nursing home care, if they do not have enough money to pay for themselves, the state will help up to certain limits, which may still leave relatives with extra money to find. In 'long stay' hospital care (over eight weeks) the pension is reduced to a small amount of 'pocket money' but no other charges are made. You may be entitled to help with travel expenses for visiting and should ask the hospital social worker about this.

Right of appeal

In the case of most state benefits, the rules are complicated and if you think you have been unfairly dealt with there is generally some right of appeal. In these cases it is worth seeking expert help and many citizens advice bureaux have specialised 'welfare rights workers' who can provide this.

Legal powers for compulsory care and treatment

The law has another role with regard to old people with a mental disorder. Sometimes it is necessary to over-rule their wishes in order to get them into hospital for treatment or into a place of continuing care. The Mental Health Act (MHA) of 1983 contains provision for the compulsory detention in hospital of people suffering from mental illness, if it is necessary in the interest of their own health or safety or in the interest of the safety of other people.

The Mental Health Act

Mentally ill people who are a serious risk to themselves or others may be admitted to hospital under section 2 (28 days) or section 3 (initially 6 months) of the MHA. A section 2 order is intended for assessment, so that doctors and others can arrive at a proper idea of what illness is present and other important factors in helping the patient. Section 3 is intended for treatment.

Mental Health Act 1983

To have someone admitted to hospital under a section 2 or 3 order you need an application by a specially trained, approved social worker (or the legally defined next of kin) and medical recommendations from two doctors. At least one of these doctors must have previous knowledge of the patient (usually the family doctor) and at least one must have special experience in the management of mental illness (usually the consultant psychiatrist). In exceptional circumstances, someone can be detained in hospital for 72 hours on the basis of an application and a single medical recommendation.

Special problem of dementia

These provisions were originally designed for people with mental illnesses such as schizophrenia, depression, and hypomania, which usually respond to medical treatment. They do not easily lend themselves to the management of people suffering from dementia, where conventional medical treatment may be of little benefit and where risks develop so slowly that it is often hard for even experienced doctors and social workers to decide when risks to safety outweigh the possible benefits of keeping the patient at home.

97

Mrs Brown was the 72 year old common law wife of an old man who had looked after her for some years until he died. Before his death, neighbours noted that she was a little 'odd' and after his death it became increasingly obvious that she was demented. Despite expert help from social services, she remained at risk in the community, largely because she did not recognise or accept the need for any help. Things came to a head one weekend when she suddenly became more confused and was unable to light her gas fire: in trying to turn it on, she somehow broke the gas pipe. Fortunately the neighbours smelled gas and called the police and gas board, who managed to get into the house and cut off the gas.

Mrs Brown would not admit that anything was wrong. Her family doctor thought that the most likely cause of the sudden increase in confusion was underlying dementia made worse by an acute confusional state caused by a urine infection.

Mrs Brown was unable to cooperate with treatment for this at home and refused hospital admission. She was admitted under section 2 of the MHA in order to sort out her immediate problems.

Guardianship order

Often, however, when a demented person is so much at risk that they need compulsory care in a safe place, they may not be so ill or severely disabled that hospital care is needed. In this case a guardianship order under the MHA may be more appropriate. Like a section 3 order, this requires an application and two medical recommendations. In this case, however, it does not allow admission to hospital, but the appointment of a guardian, who must be approved by the local social services. This guardian has three main powers. These are:

- To compel the patient to live in a specified place
- To compel the patient to attend for 'treatment' (this may for example, include appropriate day care but does *not* include the power to insist the patient actually accepts the treatment)
- To require the patient to let helping personnel such as community nurses etc into his or her home.

Advantages and disadvantages

This section of the MHA has the advantage of being less restrictive than sections 2 and 3 but has the disadvantage that the social services must be prepared to accept the responsibility of guardianship either directly through one of their employees or indirectly through the supervision of a guardian approved by them. Some social services authorities have been reluctant to accept this power, though its use is likely to increase in the future.

13 Who can help?

Sometimes relatives of dementia sufferers are tempted to despair. The help available seems so inadequate compared with the practical and emotional problems they face that there is a temptation to 'give up'. Yet relatives rarely give up so their sense of obligation often leads them to do far more than could reasonably be expected. In order to improve help to dementia sufferers and their carers, it is necessary to mount a concerted campaign for better services. Often local doctors, nurses, social workers and others will be only too well aware of the shortage of resources for this uncomplaining group. They want to improve things but find it difficult to make progress in these times of strict financial control.

Voluntary organisations can often provide practical help. They can advise about other help available and they can campaign for change. Later in this chapter there is a list of voluntary organisations that may have local branches. Usually an approach to the national office is all that is needed to find out about area branches.

Don't be afraid to complain

Remember that your own family doctor, local social services and psychiatric service for old people may often be able to do a great deal to help; but if they cannot do not be afraid to complain to the local health or social services authority. Sometimes, especially when sufferers are in long stay residential or hospital care, you may find it hard to complain about standards of care when you can see the staff are overworked and doing their best. You should not be afraid: the dementia sufferers cannot complain on their own behalf – if they do it will be dismissed as irrational – so someone has to do their complaining for them!

List of voluntary organisations that can help

Age Concern, 60 Pitcairn Road, Mitcham, Surrey CR4 3LL (01 640 5431). Produces many information packages. Has local branches some of which run sitting schemes, day centres, etc for confused old people.

Alzheimer's Disease Society, 158–160 Balham High Road, London SW12 9BN (01 675 6557). Relatively new but rapidly growing charity, specialises in helping people with dementia, regardless of age or exact diagnosis.

Association of Carers, 58 New Road, Chatham, Kent ME4 4QR (0634 813981/2). Broad based organisation concerned to help those caring for others.

Counsel and Care for the Elderly 16 Bonny Street, London NW1 9LR (01 485 1566) Information and advice principally on private residential care.

Cruse, Cruse House, 126 Sheen Road, Richmond, Surrey TW9 1UR (01 940 4818). Helps bereaved people. Has specially trained counsellors in some areas.

Disablement Income Group, Attlee House, 28 Commercial Street, London E1 6LR (01 247 2128). Special advice on benefits for disabled people and how to claim them.

Help the Aged, St James's Walk, London EC1R OBE (01 253 0253) Mostly raises funds for other charities' work with old people.

MIND (National Association for Mental Health), 22 Harley Street, London W1N 2ED (01 637 0741). Campaigns on behalf of all mentally ill people regardless of age. Many local branches run self help groups, etc. Does not specialise in old people.

Limited List
These are only a selection of the relevant national charities – usually with local branches. A fuller list can be found in *Dementia and Mental Illness in the Old* (see reading list). Your family doctor, citizens advice bureau, or social services office may have a more complete list of what is available locally.

Court of Protection

Another useful address for information on legal arrangements for the finances of mentally ill old people is The Court of Protection, 25 Store Street, London WC1E 7BP (01 636 6877). This is an ancient legal body which originally protected the interests of mentally incapacitated people with considerable financial resources. Now much of its work is to do with demented old people of more modest means.

Reading list

Home Life: a code of practice for residential care, Centre for Policy on Ageing, London 1984. This report of a DHSS sponsored working party sets out detailed standards for residential care. Many of the points made apply with equal force to nursing home and long stay hospital care. The report was endorsed by the DHSS

Living well into old age, King's Fund Project Paper 63, King Edward's Hospital Fund for London, London, 1986. This is a useful if somewhat idealistic consideration of the underpinning principles of care provision for people with dementia.

Dementia, Maurice Fraser, John Wiley & Sons, 1987. This is a fairly technical book which gives an account of recent research as well as practical approaches to the care of those suffering from dementia. It has a very positive approach and stresses how much can be done to alleviate suffering and reduce handicap in dementia sufferers even in the present state of knowledge. *Only* for those who want a detailed account of basic research as well as practice.

24-hour Approach to the problems of confusion in elderly people, Una Holden, Carol Martin, and Margaret White, Winslow Press, 1982. This booklet is available only in packs of ten but is an ideal introduction to the essential principles of daily care for the confused old person.

Reality orientation, Una Holden and Robert Woods, Churchill Livingstone, London 1982. A guide to psychological approaches to the confused elderly, this describes a compassionate and thoughtful approach to caring for those suffering from dementia. It is quite technical but not inaccessible.

The 36-hour day, Nancy Mace and Peter Rabins, Age Concern and Winslow Press, London, 1986. Highly recommended book written from the carers point of view. Looks at all the problems of caring for a dementia sufferer in the family – doesn't pull any punches!

103

Dementia and mental illness in the old, Elaine Murphy, Papermac, London 1986. Written mainly for relatives of dementia sufferers, this has more space than the present account and goes into more detail on many topics.

Managing common problems with the elderly confused, Graham Stokes, Winslow Press, Bicester 1986–7. A series of four books each dealing with a particular topic – *Wandering, Shouting and screaming, Aggression, Incontinence, and Inappropriate urinating*. Written from the psychological point of view. Simple and very helpful.

Practical psychiatry of old age, John Wattis and Mike Church, Croom Helm, London, 1986. Covers the whole of old age psychiatry from a medical and psychological viewpoint. Written for all disciplines working in old age psychiatry; does not assume any special knowledge of medicine or psychology in the reader.

More is available

This list is also highly selected. Much more is available but the books above have been chosen for their practical and realistic approach to dealing with confusion in old people.

Postscript

If you have read this book so far, you are almost certainly involved in the care of at least one confused old person. It is a demanding task, particularly if the sufferer is someone who is close to you. But it is also immensely worthwhile. In affirming the rights of those suffering from dementia to be treated as full human beings, we affirm our own humanity. This booklet aims to help you understand and deal effectively with some of the problems of caring, though nothing can substitute for human support from professionals and other carers. The booklet has at times been critical of the help offered to demented old people in this country. Many people are working very hard, however, to improve things. Unfortunately sufferers from dementia cannot shout for themselves, so it is up to us to not only to provide the care we can but to campaign for more resources to offer sufferers and their carers a fairer deal.

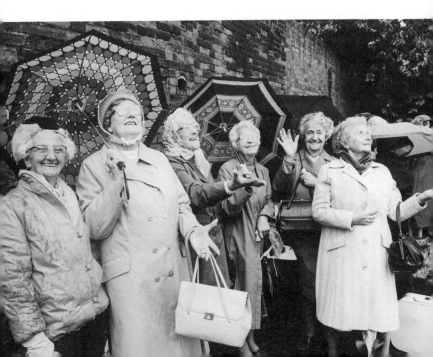

Index